Meridian Circuit Systems
A Channel Based Approach
To Pattern Identification

James Spears M.S.

Integrative Healing Press

Integrative Healing Press a Division of:
The Integrative Healing Society

Contact:
james.spears@ihsociety.com
www.ihsociety.com

ISBN: 978-1-4537842-0-4
Copyright © (2010) James Spears

Library of Congress Control Number: 2010913073

Printed in the United States of America by CreateSpace
Bulk purchases, please contact james.spears@ihsociety.com

"When you have fully grasped the principles of the three yin and three yang channels, you will then know which channel and organ is the primary and which is the secondary, and you will be able to translate the transmutations of disease among the channels."

Neijing, Chapter 79

Table of Contents

Abbreviations Used in This Book

LU – Lung

LI – Large Intestine

ST – Stomach

SP – Spleen

HT – Heart

SI – Small Intestine

UB – Urinary Bladder

KI – Kidneys

PC – Pericardium

SJ – San Jiao/Triple Warmer

GB – Gallbladder

LV – Liver

RN – Conception Meridian

DU – Governor Meridian

LK – Ling Ku

DB – Da Bai

INTRODUCTION

A meridian based approach to acupuncture therapy seems like a standard necessity; however, the most common forms of pattern identification are not based on methods that emphasize the associations between the channels. While selecting meridians and points are part of any treatment strategy, emphasis is first placed on syndrome differentiation, and secondly on determining appropriate channels and points. This is a core foundation of Chinese medicine that allows acupuncturists to address root imbalances that underlie symptomatic expressions.

If we examine the most popular methods of syndrome differentiation we will find that they are based on symptoms that are grouped according to exogenous factors, the 5-elements, or the zang-fu organs. Although it is common to identify symptoms along meridians, it is less common to actually base pattern identification on a method that works almost exclusively with the relationships that exist between the channels. For instance, if a patient suffers from a headache in the temples one may conclude that the GB meridian is involved. After this it is common for the clinician to think in terms of zang-fu or 5-element imbalances; the headache may be identified as a liver yang pattern, or an excess of fire or wind, and this depends on what other symptoms are present. It is less common for the clinician to think in terms of the temple headache as being a symptomatic expression in the foot shao yang channel, and then arriving at a treatment strategy that is based on the GB meridians connection to the SJ, LV, and HT channels.

Though a clinician that uses zang-fu or 5-element methods of differentiation may ultimately use some of the same channels, their process of determining these meridians is different than someone that uses a channel based approach to pattern identification. The meridian based approaches that I speak of have been cited by several sources including the Nei Jing, the Shang Han Lun, Dr. Richard Tan, Master Tung, and Dr. Wei-Chei Young.

A channel based approach to acupuncture takes as its starting point the relationships that exist between the meridians according to their classical Chinese names, such as the connection between the hand and foot tai yang channels. Meridian based approaches also utilize the horary cycle, and recognize not only the time designations, but also the way in which qi moves sequentially through the circuit of the twelve regular meridians.

As we progress through the pages of this book we shall learn how a meridian based approach to syndrome differentiation coincides with conventional methods of pattern identification, and is grounded in the same theory that applies to the whole of Chinese medicine. We shall also find in this analysis that meridian systems theory is able to account for many of the enigmas in Chinese medicine, as well as offer solutions to some of the most challenging cases we encounter in clinic.

One such challenge is the frequency of patients with complex patterns. Unraveling the all too common cases that simultaneously have three or more patterns presents the clinician with many technical difficulties; namely, getting the client results before they give up on the treatments. With cases that present with multiple patterns it can be extremely difficult to determine the best course of action to take. Do we treat the root, the branch, or both, and how do we get the patient the quickest and most long lasting results?

After using a meridian based approach to syndrome differentiation and treatment for many years, I have found that this method helps to clearly define the most pertinent patterns of disharmony that are present.

As clinicians our primary responsibility is getting the patient results. As we progress through our diagnostic procedures we should remember that our client did not come in to be treated for liver qi stagnation overacting on the spleen and causing dampness and blood deficiency. They came in to be treated for their condition. Though it is vitally important to do proper pattern identification, the clinician must be careful not to be overly subjective in their analysis and questioning of the patient. For it is all too common for doctors to fall into their own subjective patterns, and arrive at a conclusion of 'liver qi stagnation,' without adequately understanding what is really going on.

The clinician's inherent subjectivity often first reveals itself during the intake, and this often occurs by the way in which patients are questioned. As a result the clinician may actually unconsciously end up leading the patient into the doctor's personal favorite box of pattern identification. I don't know how many knees have been identified and treated as a kidney deficiency, yet left the patient still hobbling off with knee pain, but I can assure you this is all too common.

To assist the clinician in overcoming their own subjective tendencies I have found it crucial to ask the patient to prioritize their symptoms. A precise method for this has been developed and elaborated upon in chapter four, and it fits perfectly with the meridian based approach to pattern identification and treatment we will be discussing. When this system is employed it greatly assist in identifying patterns and developing precise treatment strategies.

Lastly, the techniques presented here are easily incorporated into all the common methods of syndrome differentiation that are used throughout the large body of Oriental medicine. Meridian systems theory integrates precisely with zang-fu, 5-elements, 8 principles, and all the other conventional methods of pattern identification. In addition, and more importantly, these methods will help any clinician to achieve greater clinical results and efficiency with fewer needles.

It is my greatest pleasure to present you with material that will better serve you and your clients needs.

CHAPTER 1

A WORLD OF PATTERNS

Essential to effective acupuncture therapy is proper pattern identification. In Chinese medicine there are at least 10 methods one may use, with the most common of these being eight principles, zang-fu, five-elements, and the six exogenous factors. While each of these represents a unique system there is also a great deal of overlap between them.

In practice many clinicians will alternate from system to system to gather all the information they need to arrive at a final diagnosis. For instance, one may arrive at the conclusion using 8 principles that a patient suffers from a condition of internal-excessive heat. Upon further examination this can be clarified using zang-fu methods to arrive at a pattern identification of liver fire. Similarly, one may determine that a patient suffers from a lung condition, but then use 8 principles to reach further clarification about the syndrome that is present. The inter-relationships that exist between the various methods of syndrome differentiation point to a universality of Chinese medical theory and practice.

Though each of the conventional methods of syndrome differentiation has been finely developed, it could be said that none of the current models represent a method of pattern identification that is primarily based in a meridian systems theory. Zang-fu differentiation is based on the patterns unique to each of the organs, and the interactions between the organ systems. Five-elements depends on the expression of the elements within the body, while six levels accounts for the various stages of cold invasions. While each of these is complete in their own right, none of them take the relationships between the 12 meridians as a focal point for identifying patterns. That is to say, none of the traditional methods of syndrome differentiation takes a meridian based perspective as a starting point. Instead, the functions and relationships of the meridians are assessed after a pattern has been identified. For instance, only after it has been determined that the patient's abdominal pain is due to liver qi stagnation, rather than other possible patterns, will the meridians and points be selected. This is essential to traditional methods of differentiation because the clinician needs to know what the diagnosis is before developing a treatment strategy.

There are however methods to determine patterns and treatments that are based primarily on meridian relationships. These methods are discussed by Dr. Richard Tan and are a fundamental aspect of Tung style acupuncture as well. The basic concept of these systems is to identify what meridians are expressing symptoms, and then determine what connecting meridians may be used to treat the condition. For a condition like knee pain, a meridian systems method will first determine precisely what meridian is affected, and then decide what meridians should be used to treat it. If the pain is located on the ST channel, it is likely that the LI meridian would be chosen for treatment since the LI connects to the ST through the yang ming.

This method of identifying patterns and developing treatments based on meridian connections and associations is much different than traditional methods such as zang-fu and 5-elements. In the above example of knee pain, it would be common for someone practicing zang-fu differentiation to start to look for other signs or symptoms that would confirm a kidney pattern. This method has limitations in actual practice because there are numerous causes to knee pain besides kidney deficiency. In a meridian based approach we are primarily concerned with what meridians are expressing symptoms.

Symptomatic Meridians and Their Connections

A meridian systems approach to pattern identification and treatment takes as its starting point the meridian that is symptomatically affected, and the meridians that are connected to it. To begin to understand ways in which the meridians are associated with one another we need to start with the six meridian pairs as classified in the six stages of syndrome differentiation. These are expounded upon in the Shang Han Lun and include the six pairs of tai yang, yang ming, shao yang, tai yin, shao yang, and jue yin. Though the Shang Han Lun discusses these meridians in the context of external cold invasions, this method of pairing the meridians is based on yin-yang relationships, anatomical location, and physiological functions. Taking the yang ming pair as an example we find that it contains one hand meridian and one foot meridian. Additionally, these meridians are located on the most anterior yang portions of the body, and they share functions in digestive processes. Similarly, the shao yin pair includes one hand and foot meridian, and these are located on the most posterior yin aspects of the body. In terms of functionality the shao yin govern the most vital fluids of the body, namely the blood and essence. We shall examine these

3

relationships further in chapter two, but for now it is important to recognize that the six meridians are one way in which meridians may be paired together.

Another way the meridians may be paired is through what is called the Zang Fu Bei Tong Theory. This way of pairing meridians is a major component of Tung style acupuncture, and is referred to as the system two associations in Dr. Tan's methods. This system takes the tai yang meridians and pairs them with the tai yin, and draws a relationship between the foot tai yang (UB) and the hand tai yin (LU), and between the hand tai yang (SI) and the foot tai yin (SP). Similarly, the shao yang meridians are associated with the shao yin, and the yang ming are paired with the jue yin. It is through this system that the LI and LV meridians form a connection, and this relationship is most commonly recognized in the point combination of LI 4 and LV 3.

The meridians may also be joined based on their internal/external relationships. These types of pairs are well known and include the LU – LI connection as well as the KI – UB pair.

Meridians may also be grouped according to the horary cycle. In this system each of the twelve regular meridians have a designated two hour period of time during a 24-hour day. There are two ways to pair meridians based on the horary cycle, and we shall elaborate on these in the next chapter.

These relationships that exist between the meridians are recognized in various contexts and form the foundation of Master Tung and Dr. Tan's methods. However, these systems of connection between the meridians are something that has not been adequately explored by the larger Chinese medical community. These systems do however deserve careful attention due their ability to quickly resolve disease patterns with the use of fewer needles.

A New Method for Identifying Patterns

The methods presented herein represent a unique form of syndrome differentiation that may be used independently of other methods. It may also be used to assist in conventional forms of pattern identification and it can greatly assist the clinician in determining zang-fu patterns. Meridian systems theory takes as its starting point the identification of meridians that are expressing symptoms, and then determines the relationship the affected meridian shares with other channels. After the symptomatic meridians and their connecting channels have been established, meridian systems theory aims at identifying a circuit that consists of four meridians that are inter-connected. A four meridian (4M) circuit is then identified to determine the primary pattern that is responsible for the patient's chief symptoms. We shall elaborate on this in chapter five but for now let's continue our discussion of how syndromes are recognized.

Any system of syndrome differentiation is based on two things, the underlying theory, and symptomatic patterns that define the syndrome. Therefore, a new method of pattern identification needs to be in agreement with the established knowledge that Chinese medicine holds to be true, and it would also need to be able to recognize and define patterns of disharmony that are repeatedly observable in clinical practice. The final measure of a new system of syndrome differentiation rests unequivocally in its ability to produce clinical results.

5

As we build the foundation of using meridian systems theory for syndrome differentiation, we will use the established knowledge of Chinese medicine. This will include classical sources such as the Nei Jing, the Hang Shan Lun, 5-element theory, as well as knowledge from TCM, Master Tung, and Dr. Richard Tan.

Meridian systems theory is then an integration of the various methods that we have come to know as the large body of Chinese medicine. It is not meant to replace or undermine any of the traditional methods of syndrome differentiation; rather, it will assist the clinician in identifying patterns of disharmony and developing more precise treatment strategies. This system can be incorporated into any style of practice, and it will greatly assist the clinician in achieving greater therapeutic results.

As a final note, meridian systems theory provides answers and clarification to many of the mysteries that exist in the conventional teachings on acupuncture. From better understanding of point indications, to recognizing patterns in the 5-shu points, meridian systems theory guides the precision of needlework to the next level.

CHAPTER 2

THE FIVE SYSTEMS

The systems that are a fundamental part of meridian systems theory have been described by several classical and traditional sources. For simplicity I have adopted Dr. Richard Tan's notation of the five systems as it is highly organized, well known, and lends itself to easy descriptions once the systems are learned. We shall now briefly describe the five systems before elaborating on the theoretical and clinical applications of them.

System 1

The first system is referred to as the six meridians of tai yang, yang ming, shao yang, tai yin, shao yin, and jue yin. These divisions have a long history and are spoken of extensively in the Nei Jing and the Shang Han Lun. Although commonly known in the six stages of syndrome differentiation these pairs have broad applications in many other contexts as well. We shall cover this in a later section but for now let's review the system one pairs.

Tai Yang: SI – UB	Shao Yang: SJ – GB	Yang Ming: LI – ST
Tai Yin: LU – SP	Shao Yin: HT – KI	Jue Yin: LV – PC

7

System 2

The system two associations are also known as the Zang Fu Bei Tong theory. This system has its origins in two Ming Dynasty texts the *Yi Xie Ru Men* and the *Yi Jin Jin Yi*. In this system the tai yang are associated with the tai yin to create a correspondence between the urinary bladder and lung, a similar relationship is also established between the small intestine and spleen. The shao yang is associated with the shao yin in such a way that the heart pairs with the gallbladder, and the kidneys pair with the san jiao. Similarly, the yang ming is paired with the jue yin so that the stomach and pericardium form a pair, and the large intestine and liver form a connection as well. These associations are represented as:

Tai Yang: UB - SI	Shao Yang: GB - SJ	Yang Ming: LI - ST
Tai Yin: LU - SP	Shao Yin: HT - KI	Jue Yin: LV - PC

System 3

System three is well known as the internal-external relationships that exist between the meridians. This is a fundamental teaching in all styles of acupuncture, and since this system is so well known we will not spend much time discussing it now. The system three connections are listed in the table at the end of this section.

System 4

System four is based on the horary cycle that relates a two-hour period of time to each meridian. In this system a correspondence is recognized between meridians at opposite sides of the clock. For instance, the time from 11:00 am - 1:00 pm is recognized as heart time, and 11:00 pm - 1:00 am is classified as gallbladder time. System four pairs the heart and gallbladder based on their positions opposite of one another on the clock. This is done for each of the meridians and forms the following pairs:

LU – UB	LI – KI	ST – PC	SP – SJ	HT – GB	SI – LV

System 5

This system pairs the meridians that are located next to each other on the clock that have the same yin-yang classification. In this system the spleen and heart are paired because they are located next to each other, spleen time is from 9:00 am - 11:00 am, and the heart's time is 11:00 am - 1:00 pm. The system 5 pairs are:

LU – LV	LI – ST	SP – HT	SI – UB	KI – PC	GB – SJ

The five systems for each meridian are presented on the next page.

5 Systems Chart

	1	2	3	4	5
LU	SP	UB	LI	UB	LV
LI	ST	LV	LU	KI	ST
ST	LI	PC	SP	PC	LI
SP	LU	SI	ST	SJ	HT
HT	KI	GB	SI	GB	SP
SI	UB	SP	HT	LV	UB
UB	SI	LU	KI	LU	SI
KI	HT	SJ	UB	SJ	PC
PC	LV	ST	SJ	ST	KI
SJ	GB	KI	PC	SP	GB
GB	SJ	HT	LV	HT	SJ
LV	PC	LI	GB	SI	LU

The Five Systems and Chinese Medical Theory

The following sections will compare the five meridian systems to traditional theories and applications and show that there is much in common between them. Through doing this we will find that meridian systems theory concurs with established theories and practices of Chinese medicine, and even provides additional insight on point functions and standard treatment protocols.

We shall begin our discussion with the system one associations that are also known as the six meridians. These will not be reviewed in the context of the six stages of cold invasion as taught in the Shang Han Lun but in terms of shared functional activity.

The Tai Yang Meridians of the Small Intestine and Urinary Bladder

Functions:

1) Circulates qi through the tai yang channels and the eyes, head, neck, back, shoulders, and spine.

2) Distributes wei qi to the most exterior regions of the body.

3) Regulates fluid metabolism through the functions of the small intestine and bladder.

The tai yang meridians are strongly associated with the head, eyes, neck, back, shoulders, and spine. This is apparent by the location of the meridians, as well as SI 3's connection to the DU mai. While the tai yang meridians are connected with the yang and qi aspect of the spine and nervous system, the heart and kidneys are related to the yin aspect through the blood, essence, and marrow. This is an important distinction to make between the tai yang and the shao yin, as they are both influential in various aspects of nervous system functioning.

The tai yang meridians are also associated with the wei qi and distribute it to the most superficial regions of the body. In six stages, the tai yang are usually the first meridians invaded by external cold pathogens. It is also important to consider the connection between the tai yang and tai yin when considering conditions related to the immune system. The tai yang functions to circulate the wei qi through the exterior of the body, while the tai yin has a strong association with the anti-pathogenic qi.

The tai yang also have important functions in regards to fluid metabolism. Basic theory teaches us that both the

11

small intestine and bladder regulate the fluids. The small intestine separates the pure from the impure, and sends the impure fluids to the urinary bladder for excretion. The role of the tai yang in regulating fluid metabolism and excretion is another function that connects the tai yang and the tai yin.

The Yang Ming Meridians of the Large Intestine and Stomach

Functions:

1) Regulates the stomach and intestines.

2) Influences digestion.

3) Harmonizes the bowels.

The yang ming connection between the LI and ST meridians is one of the most widely utilized system one associations. On the ST meridian we find many points that influence the large intestine. Stomach 25 is the front-mu point, ST 36 is well known for treating bowel conditions, and ST 37 is the lower he-sea point of the large intestine. On the large intestine meridian we find that LI 10 is energetically similar to ST 36, and there are numerous other points on the large intestine that are capable of treating various stomach and abdominal conditions.

The Shao Yang Meridians of the San Jiao and Gallbladder

Functions:

1) Distributes qi through the shao yang channels including the head, neck, shoulders, and ribcage.

2) Opens the Yang Wei and Dai mai meridians.

3) Resolves wind.

4) Regulates water passages.

The shao yang meridians are well known as a pair and are often used together through the use of GB 41 and SJ 5. These two points in combination open the Dai mai and Yang Wei meridians. The Yang Wei, which is opened by SJ 5, has many crossing points with the gallbladder meridian including GB 35 and GB 13 - GB 20. For this reason SJ 5 is indicated for treating temple headaches and neck pain, and this reveals one way in which the SJ may be used to treat the GB meridian. Similarly, various acupuncture sources cite SJ 4 as having the effect of draining GB 20 and opening the neck.

Due to the shao yang's location along the head and neck it has a strong connection to the nervous system. The shao yang meridians are especially helpful for treating liver yang rising, internal wind, as well as certain mental-emotional conditions. We shall expand on this in a later section when we examine the connection the shao yang shares with both the shao yin and the jue yin, but for now it is enough to recognize that the shao yang are indicated for difficult conditions that affect the nervous system such as internal wind and liver yang rising.

The Tai Yin Meridians of the Spleen and Lungs

Functions:

1) Governs qi through respiration and digestion.

2) Regulates water and fluid metabolism.

3) Influences the anti-pathogenic qi.

The tai yin meridians share the functions of governing qi and regulating water metabolism. While the lungs govern qi and respiration, the spleen governs the post-natal qi. Taken together we may say that the lungs and spleen play a primary role in replenishing qi through respiration and digestion. If we look at the Chinese character for qi we find that it is composed of two radicals, one representing vapor, and the other representing rice. The vapor component represents the air that we breathe and the rice radical represents food.

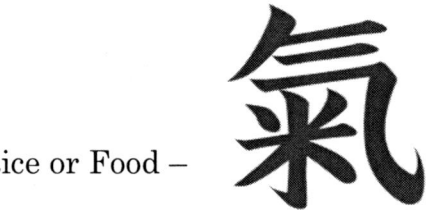

Rice or Food –   – Vapor or Air

The character for qi then represents the raw energy that is contained in air and food, and as we know from physiology these are the basic substances that supply us with energy. For these reasons the tai yin plays a primary role in replenishing qi, and whenever qi deficiency exists the relative function of the tai yin should be assessed.

The tai yin organs also play a major role in water metabolism. Physiology teaches that the lungs regulate the water passages by sending fluids to the urinary bladder and kidneys, while the spleen is responsible for the transformation and transportation of dampness. Therefore, the lungs disperse and descend fluids, while the spleen functions with the digestive system to metabolize and process water. This joint function of metabolizing fluids is a major activity of the tai yin.

The tai yin meridians of the lungs and spleen have the joint functions of governing qi and regulating the movement and transformation of fluids. For this reason, when we observe patterns involving qi deficiency, and/or fluid metabolism, we must consider the interrelated functions of the tai yin organs. It is often helpful in clinical situations to view the organs of the spleen and lungs functioning together as the tai yin pair.

The Shao Yin Meridians of the Heart and Kidneys

Functions:

1) Governs the blood and essence.

2) Harmonizes yin-yang dynamics.

3) Regulates fire and water balance.

The shao yin meridians share the function of governing the most vital fluids of the body. The heart governs the blood, and the kidneys govern the essence. The shao yin also plays a major role in regulating yin-yang dynamics since they are connected to the primary elements of water and fire. The kidneys govern water, store essence, produce marrow, and are the source of the ming men fire. Their role in regulating yin-yang, and maintaining proper water and fire balance, is closely coordinated with the heart functions of governing blood and housing the spirit.

The yang and fire components of the heart and kidneys are a primary way in which yang is distributed throughout the entire body. While the heart distributes fire energy through the circulation of the blood, the yuan qi from the kidneys is distributed through the body via the san jiao. In regards to the yin of the heart and kidneys, physiology teaches that the blood and essence share the same source. This demonstrates the deep connection that exists between the heart and kidneys as pertains to the most vital fluids and elements of the body.

The Jue Yin Meridians of the Liver and Gallbladder

Functions:

1) Regulates circulation of qi and blood.

2) Calms the spirit.

3) Supplements yin and blood.

The jue yin meridians play a major role in the circulation of qi and blood. Chinese medical theory teaches that the liver maintains the free flow of qi, and the pericardium functions with the heart to circulate the blood. Therefore, these two organs are connected by way of their function in controlling and regulating the circulation of the qi and blood.

Physiology also teaches that the liver stores blood, and the connections between the liver and pericardium are further defined by each of these organs relationship with the blood. The liver regulates blood storage but depends on the functions of the pericardium to move it.

The jue yin also has strong connections to the spirit, and we most easily observe this in the functions of the liver and pericardium points. While the pericardium points help to calm the spirit and regulate the emotions, the liver meridian is very useful for clearing stagnant emotions, releasing irritability, and calming the mind.

In clinic we can easily observe how the liver is one of the first organs that is affected by stress, and when mental and emotional stress is present it often manifests through liver signs and symptoms. Due to the connection between the liver and pericardium, as well as the pericardium's ability to resolve liver stagnation, it is common to use pericardium points when the liver is adversely affected by emotional

17

factors. The pericardium's function of protecting the heart also establishes it as a primary meridian for treating conditions of the mind and emotions.

One of the functions of PC 6 is to move qi and resolve liver stagnation. It is useful for anxiety caused by liver qi stagnation, as well as various menstrual conditions that are rooted in liver imbalances. In addition, PC 6 may also be used for situations where the liver is adversely affecting the stomach. From shen disturbance, to menstrual conditions and abdominal complaints, we find that the pericardium meridian is useful for a variety of symptoms that have an underlying liver imbalance.

System 2 Connections

The Lungs and Urinary Bladder: LU – UB

One of the functions of the lungs is to regulate water metabolism by sending fluids to the kidneys and urinary bladder. In system two we find a connection between the lung and bladder meridians, and the most well known connection between these channels is the use of LU 7 to treat the back of the neck. This point is usually indicated when the neck is affected by wind-cold invasions and tai yang syndrome.

To expand our clinical use of LU 7 it may be used for any condition of the neck when the UB meridian is affected. Regardless of etiology or diagnosis, LU 7 may be used to treat the neck when symptoms are present in the UB channel. This point is best utilized when the symptoms are located from UB 10 to UB 13.

Another example of how LU 7 may be used to treat conditions of the urinary bladder, occur by way of LU 7 being the opening point of the RN meridian. The RN meridian begins in the lower abdomen and passes through the region of the bladder. At the beginning of the RN meridian is the bladder, and near the terminal portion of the RN are the lungs and respiratory system. The Ren mai is the extra-ordinary meridian that connects these two organs, and for this reason, LU 7 is a good choice for conditions that affect the bladder.

In addition to the effects of LU 7 on the bladder, we also find that LU 5 is the water point on the lung meridian. This being the case we should find that LU 5 has an effect on the bladder, and in fact, many acupuncture sources state that LU 5 benefits the UB and helps to descend water flow. The point is also indicated for water accumulation and low back pain. In addition, LU 5 is energetically similar to UB 40, and they both are beneficial for low back pain and regulating water metabolism. Building on this correspondence we find that UB 40 is indicated for various skin conditions such as rashes and itching. Since the lungs are connected to the skin, we find yet another association between these two meridians.

Diseases of the Bladder

Lung 5 and LU 7 may be used in combination for all types of conditions that involve the urinary bladder. Other points along the LU meridian will also effect the UB meridian, but for actual diseases of the bladder organ the LU 5 and LU 7 combination is superior. For acute and excessive conditions, or when blood is present in the urine, it can also be helpful to add LU 6, the xi-cleft point.

Upper Back Pain

Ashi points located between LU 6 and LU 7 are very effective for treating upper back pain when it is located along the bladder channel. Palpation along the lung meridian should be done to find the most sensitive points, and when needling strong qi sensation should be obtained. Points may be needled on either side, and teach the client to apply self-massage to the points 2-3 times a day.

The Large Intestine and Liver: LI – LV

The large intestine – liver pair is a well known system two connection, as four gates is one of the most widely used point combinations in acupuncture. This combination is indicated for qi stagnation, blood stagnation, pain, shen disturbance, and many other things. Although there are few explanations why this large intestine – liver pairing is so powerful, we can see that meridian systems theory provides a way to understand the relationship between these channels.

Another explanation for the effectiveness of four gates is that metal overacts on wood, and by needling LI 4 we are strongly moving the qi of the liver.

Regardless of what theory we use to understand the usefulness of this point combination, we should recognize that meridian systems theory gives us a method to integrate and better understand the various models and theories of Oriental medicine.

The Stomach and Pericardium: ST – PC

The stomach and pericardium pair are commonly used in clinic whenever PC 6 is used to treat abdominal and stomach conditions. It is well known that PC 6 harmonizes the stomach, and combines well with a number of stomach points to treat digestive and abdominal complaints. Lesser known is the use of PC 3 for stomach and abdominal conditions, but many acupuncture sources list PC 3 as having the energetic function of regulating the stomach and intestines. The ability of PC 3 to regulate the stomach and abdomen comes from its system two correspondence with the stomach.

Pericardium 3 and 6 are a powerful point combination to use for a wide variety of stomach and abdominal complaints, I have even found that applying pressure to these points will often stop nausea, bloating, and abdominal discomfort within minutes. For a wide variety of digestive and abdominal conditions use PC 3 and PC 6 in combination with the appropriate ST meridian points.

The Spleen and Small Intestine: SP – SI

The spleen and small intestine connection is one that is often overlooked and rarely utilized in clinic. In theory we find numerous connections between these organs in both physiology and 5-element models. According to 5-elements, the SI is a fire channel and may be used to strengthen the earth energy. In Chinese medical theory the small intestine functions to separate the clear and turbid fluids, while the spleen is responsible for the transformation and transportation of the fluids. Both of these organs are important for water metabolism.

The Heart and Gallbladder: HT – GB

This is an association that is well known in Chinese medicine, and in zang-fu pattern terminology is referred to as a heart and gallbladder deficiency. This pattern has characteristic symptoms such as lack of courage, inability to make decisions, and other heart and liver/gallbladder symptoms. Though this pattern may not be very common in clinic, the important thing for now is to recognize that the heart – gallbladder connection is spoken of in terms of a zang-fu syndrome.

When using the correspondence between the heart and gallbladder in meridian systems theory, we are not necessarily looking for the symptoms that define a heart and gallbladder deficiency. Rather, we are using the gallbladder channel to treat conditions affecting the heart meridian, and vice a versa, the heart channel is employed to treat conditions involving the gallbladder meridian.

For pain in the GB channel along the path between GB 20 - GB 21 use HT 4, HT 5, and/or Ht 7. Heart 4 is located 1.5 cun above the wrist crease and is at the same level as Lu 7. While Lu 7 is most appropriate to use when the neck symptoms are in the UB channel, the heart points are more effective for patterns manifesting in the GB channel.

When pain is located in the neck and shoulders between GB 20 - GB 21 it is often related to stress and tension that is common in type A personalities. The use of HT 4, HT 5, and HT 7 not only has the effect of influencing the GB meridian, but these points also function to calm the mind and are very useful when stress is a contributing factor to neck and shoulder symptoms.

The Kidneys and San Jiao: KI – SJ

The connection between the kidneys and san jiao is very well known. Traditional theory teaches that the san jiao distributes kidney yang throughout the body and acts as a water passageway. The fire component of the triple warmer is derived from the kidney yang, and without the original fire from the kidneys the san jiao would not be able to perform its function of distributing yuan qi through the body.

San jiao points may be used to clear heat from the body, treat constipation, and resolve internal wind, and each of these conditions correlates with its connection to the kidneys. One common way that san jiao points are used that acknowledges this connection is the use of SJ 5 for clearing empty heat from the body. When the kidney yin has declined and is causing empty heat, SJ 5 is commonly indicated. Conversely, SJ 5 may be used with moxa to add heat to the body in patterns of yang deficiency. In cases of constipation, SJ 6 may be used as it effectively clears heat due to kidney yin deficiency. Similarly, the use of SJ points are indicated in cases of internal wind that are rooted in liver and kidney yin deficiencies.

System 4 Connections

For many of the meridians the system two and system four correspondences are the same. For example, the lungs and urinary bladder are connected in both system two and four. The same is also true for the pericardium and stomach, as well as the heart and gallbladder. The system four connections we will explore in this section are the ones that have not already been covered.

The Large Intestine and Kidneys: LI – KI

In system four we find a connection between the large intestine and kidneys, and there are a number of points that are widely used that acknowledge the association between these meridians.

Kidney 7 is commonly indicated for the treatment of diarrhea when there is an underlying kidney yang deficiency, and KI 6 is indicated for constipation when the yin is deficient. In both of these examples we see that the kidney meridian is able to regulate the function of the large intestine. Meridian systems theory shows us this connection exists in system four and is based on the horary cycle.

Kidney 7 is also commonly combined with LI 4 to regulate the wei qi, and this point combination can either cause or stop sweating. These points may be used for either excessive wind-cold conditions, or internal deficiency, and needle technique dictates the response.

Another major connection between the LI and KI meridians can be found in Master Tung's point Ling Ku. This point is located on the LI meridian at the junction between the first and second metacarpal joints. It is well known for its ability to treat lumbar pain, urinary diseases, and prostate conditions.

The Spleen and San Jiao: SP – SJ

This is a fire-earth association that is easily comprehended by understanding the functions of the san jiao. As we have already mentioned, the san jiao and kidneys are linked through system two, and the san jiao functions to transport yuan qi and kidney yang throughout the body. Since the spleen relies on the kidneys for yang qi, the san jiao is the avenue through which the kidney yang is transported to the spleen. Likewise, the san jiao also functions as a passage for water metabolism, and the spleen functions in the transportation and transformation of fluids. The spleen and san jiao are connected through the kidney yang and their mutual roles in fluid metabolism.

Both traditional theory and meridian systems teach that there is a connection between the SJ and SP meridians; however, this is often under-utilized in clinical practice. Keeping this in mind, we should examine the possibility of using the SJ meridian in cases where the spleen qi or yang is deficient, and when damp accumulation is impairing the functions of the spleen. Some systems of Japanese acupuncture use moxa on san jiao points in cases of spleen qi and yang deficiency, and this may be easily understood in 5-element terms as fire engenders earth.

The Small Intestine and Liver: SI – LV

The small intestine and liver correspondence is under recognized, but it is a very powerful association that has broad applications. Many acupuncture sources reference the connection between these meridians in two points, SI 4 and SI 7. Small intestine 4 is known to be an empirical point for jaundice, and it may be used to treat damp heat conditions of the liver. The luo point of the small intestine meridian, SI 7, is also known to be good for emotional patterns that involve the liver and gallbladder.

Another well known correspondence between the SI and LV occurs when SI 3 is used to treat internal wind and conditions such as epilepsy, convulsions, and tremors. Though it is usually thought that this benefit arises from SI 3 opening the DU, it is also due to this points ability to treat internal wind that is rooted in a liver imbalance.

In Master Tung's acupuncture we find two very effective points on the SI meridian that are able to regulate liver function, these are 33.11 and 33.10. Otherwise known as Liver Gate, 33.11, is located 6 cun above the pisiform bone on the SI meridian, it is indicated for acute hepatitis.

System 5 Connections

The Lungs and Liver: LU – LV

The correspondence between the LU and LV is a very powerful one that deserves special attention. In traditional theories we find that liver fire may invade the lungs, and that the metal of the lungs may overact on the liver. Through system five the LU and LV are connected because of their location next to each other on the clock, and in the sequential movement of qi through the meridians the qi moves from the LV meridian to the LU meridian at 5 a.m. This junction between the ending and beginning of a new cycle is a very important one that can be effectively applied in clinic.

When tightness of the chest occurs due to underlying liver qi stagnation, or emotional repression, using four gates in conjunction with LU 1 and LV 14 is a very effective point combination. Begin by needling LU 1 followed by LI 4, this activates the metal so that we may reduce the excess wood of the liver. After needling LI 4, needle LV 14 followed by LV 3, as needling against the meridian flow is one way to reduce an excessive condition. This combination of LU 1 and LV 14 I refer to as thoracic four gates, it is very powerful whenever liver patterns affect the upper jiao, and it is also a strong point combination for releasing stagnant emotional energy from the chest.

The Spleen and Heart: SP – HT

The connection between the spleen and heart is well known in traditional theories that teach that the spleen produces the qu qi and the heart transforms the qu qi into blood. We also find that in the regular cycle of the meridians the qi moves from the spleen to the heart meridian at 11 a.m. In terms of point indications and functions, SP 10 invigorates the circulation and production of blood and can be useful for numerous heart patterns. Spleen 6 is another important point that is widely used for heart patterns, especially when the heart yin needs to be supplemented, or if there is shen disturbance rooted in a heart imbalance. For conditions of shen disturbance SP 6 is as often used, or even more so than HT 7.

The Kidneys and Pericardium: KI – PC

In system five the KI and PC are connected because they are located next to each other on the clock. This relationship between the kidney water and heart fire is so fundamental that we find that the kidneys pair with both the HT and PC. The combination of the KI and PC meridians have broad applications in clinical practice and may be used to treat abdominal conditions, shen disturbance, liver patterns, and hormonal imbalance. We shall examine these functions in greater detail when we discuss the various circuits.

Using the Five Systems to Determine Roots and Branches

The connections between the meridians as established by the five systems can greatly assist us in determining root and branch patterns. We can understand this by observing

27

that it is common for the primarily affected meridian to manifest the branch symptom, while one of its connecting meridians is often responsible for the root pattern. Let's look at an example of how this occurs in headaches. Suppose a patient has chronic temple headaches that affect the GB channel. Reviewing the GB's connecting meridians we find the following:

GB - SJ - HT - LV - HT - SJ

Typically temple headaches are identified as a liver yang rising pattern when they occur with anger, dizziness, hypertension, and pain in the hypochondria. In system three the GB connects to the liver. Going back to our discussion of branch and root patterns we find:

Branch Symptom Affects – GB channel
Root Pattern – Liver Yang Rising

Another cause of temple headaches is blood deficiency, and this pattern may also occur with symptoms such as insomnia, palpitations, dizziness, and numbness. In this pattern blood deficiency and heart imbalances are present, and in system two and four the GB and HT are connected.

Branch Symptom Affects – GB channel
Root Pattern – Heart Blood Deficiency

Temple headaches may also be due to an external wind-heat invasion and SJ points can be chosen for this pattern.

Branch Symptom Affects – GB channel
Root Pattern – Wind Heat Invasion, use SJ points

When treating temple headaches we want to select the most appropriate meridians based on the syndrome that is present. For temple headaches due to liver yang rising we would want to choose the LV meridian as a primary channel for treatment. In cases where the patient has temple headaches with blood deficiency and heart signs, the HT meridian becomes a primary channel for treatment. If the headache is due to wind heat then the SJ channel becomes one of our first choices for treatment. Although this is a simplified example of how to choose meridians, and is in no way complete for determining final treatment strategies, it does give us an extra way of discovering root patterns of imbalance.

In some cases it is not challenging to determine root patterns, but in complex cases when multiple syndromes are present it can be difficult to identify the most important syndrome to treat. Using this method of identifying the symptomatic meridians as a branch, and its connecting meridians as possible locations for root disharmonies, is a simple and effective way to gain perspective on various conditions. Whenever there is difficulty identifying a zang-fu syndrome the five meridian systems can be used to help determine where the greatest disharmony is located. By viewing the affected meridian as a branch symptom, we can use its associated meridians in the five systems to point us in the direction of finding the root cause.

Let's look at one more example of how the meridian systems correspond with zang-fu patterns and can assist in determining root causes. This time we will consider several patterns of constipation. Constipation may or may not produce pain or symptoms along the meridians, but it is a condition that affects the large intestine, and for this reason we will take the LI meridian as our affected channel. Reviewing the five system connections for the LI we find:

LI - ST - LV - LU - KI - ST

One of the most common patterns of constipation is excessive heat, and this is often related to stomach heat. In system one the LI and ST are connected.

Branch Symptom of Constipation – LI
Root Cause – Stomach Heat, ST

For yin deficiency constipation the treatment strategy is to supplement the kidney yin, and in system four the LI and KI are connected.

Branch Symptom of Constipation – LI
Root Cause – Kidney Yin Deficiency, KI

In cases of constipation due to liver stagnation, we find a system two connection between the LI and LV.

Branch Symptom of Constipation – LI
Root Cause – Liver Qi Stagnation, LV

In each of the above cases we started with the organ or meridian that is primarily affected, and then determined meridian system correspondences and root causes. Though this method of correlating two connecting meridians to roots and branches has wide applications, it does have limitations that should be acknowledged. First of all it is not able to explain all patterns that may be possible for any symptom or disease, nor will the affected meridian connect to all the organs that may be involved in the pathogenesis. Rather, the meridian systems provide insight and direction for identifying some of the possible patterns, and they usually point to the meridians that will produce the greatest effect when treated.

Though the process of syndrome differentiation is more complex than simply determining a connecting meridian according to the five systems, the method of looking for possible root causes in the five system correspondences has numerous benefits for diagnosis and treatment. We shall continue to build on this line of thought in later chapters when we discuss the more complex fundamentals of doing syndrome differentiation based on the meridian systems.

CHAPTER 3

IMAGING, MIRRORING,
AND NEEDLING

The technique of using non-local points to treat various diseases is widely utilized in acupuncture. In fact, non-local needling is one of the fundamental practices of meridian therapy. The basic theory of acupuncture is that by needling the meridians one can influence the function of the internal organs and other systems. In Chinese medicine we also find various statements that convey the use of non-local needling such as "needle the feet to affect the head." Though there are numerous ways to understand this, meridian systems theory uses the methods of imaging and mirroring to explain a number of non-local needling techniques and responses. Let's start with the concept of imaging.

> **Imaging is defined as superimposing body images on one another to map out areas of correspondence.**

The most common form of imaging is found in the ear acupuncture systems where the whole body is mapped on the ear. Imaging is also utilized in the Korean hand systems that map the body on the hands. In regards to using the 12 regular meridians and their standard points, we find that the hands and feet image the head. This means that for conditions of the head and face we can needle the hands and/or feet. The use of LI 4 to treat sinus congestion and headaches is one example of this method.

While the hands and feet image the head, the wrist and ankles image the neck. This means we can use points along the wrist or ankles to treat the neck and throat. The use of LU 7, UB 60, GB 39, and SJ 4 for treating neck conditions conveys this principle.

As we move to the elbows and knees we find that they image the navel and upper lumbar area. So for conditions of the mid-abdominal and lumbar regions we may use points located around the elbows and knees. As examples ST 36, LI 10, UB 40, LU 5, SP 9, and PC 3 all demonstrate the functions of this imaging method.

For areas below the navel, the upper arms and thighs image the lower abdomen and lumbrosacral area, and finally the shoulders and hips image the genitals. One example of how points on the shoulder may be used to treat the reproductive system and genitals is the use of Master Tung's point Yun Bai (44.11) for treating vaginal pain, leucorrhea, and vaginitis.

The imaging methods just discussed are used extensively in Tung style acupuncture and are also widely taught by Dr. Richard Tan. Related to these imaging methods is another technique taught by Dr. Tan that images long bones to the spine and torso. In this system the distal portion of the long bones image the throat, neck, and cervical vertebrae, and the proximal portions of the long bones correspond to the abdomen, lower lumbar, and sacral areas. The images on the next page show how the spine corresponds to the long bones.

Imaging the Spine with Long Bones

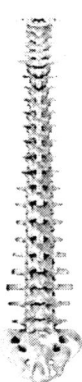

Cervical Area – Distal Portion

Lumbar Area – Proximal Portion

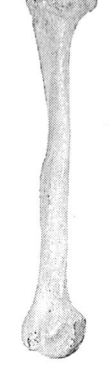

This method of imaging the spine to the long bones explains the functions of points such as GB 41, SP 4, LU 7, SI 3, UB 65, Yao Tong Xue, and Luo Zhen Xue.

Luo Zhen Xue is the pair of points located on the dorsum of the hand between the 2nd and 3rd, and the 4th and 5th metacarpals; they are located just proximal to the meta-carpophalangeal joint. This area corresponds to the distal portion of the metacarpals, and these points are known to treat stiffness in the neck. Similarly, Yao Tong Xue are a pair of points located on the dorsum of the hand between the 2nd and 3rd, and 4th and 5th metacarpals. They are located at the most proximal portions of the metacarpals and are outstanding for treating lumbar pain. These well known points support the theory that images the spine to the long bones.

Another example of this imaging method is the use of GB 41 to open the Dai mai. Remember that GB 41 is located just distal to the junction between the 4th and 5th metatarsals. Therefore, we may also say that GB41 is located at the proximal portion of the long bones of the metatarsals. Since the proximal portions of the long bones correspond to the lower abdominal and lumbar area, we find that GB 41 strongly influences these regions. A similar example may be found with SP 4 opening the Chong mai. Recall that SP 4 is located at the proximal portion of the first metatarsal, an area that corresponds with the lower abdominal and lumbar area in our imaging of the spine and torso to long bones.

For neck conditions we also find that SI 3 is located at the distal portion of the 5th metacarpal, and UB 65 at the distal portion of the 5th metatarsal. This is yet another common example of how the distal portions of the long bones correspond to the neck and cervical regions.

Returning to our theory that the hands and feet image the head, we already mentioned that LI 4 is used to treat sinus congestion and headaches. This is a very common example of using a point on the hand to treat the head and face. On the GB meridian, GB 43 is indicated for temple headaches and ear conditions, while GB 42 and GB 44 treat eye disorders. More generally, but also related to the theory of imaging the head to the hands and feet, we find that the jing-well points are indicated for treating the sensory organs of the head. This can also be understood by imaging theory that relates the head to the hands and feet.

In regards to the ankles and wrist imaging the neck, we find that LU 7 and SJ 4 are both indicated for conditions of the neck, as are UB 60, GB 39, and GB 40. Lung 7 is best used for pain in the UB meridian, because of its system two correspondence with the UB. San jiao 4 is to be used for treating the area of GB 20, and this is due to the SJ and GB pairing in system one. In regards to UB 60, it is best to use this point when the symptoms are present in the UB or SI meridians.

Moving proximally up from the wrists and ankles we find that the distal portions of the arms and legs image the thoracic area. The jing-river points located just proximal to the wrist and ankles are known to treat asthma and cough, and this once again shows us how common point indications and functions correspond to the imaging methods we are discussing.

Mirroring

Imaging and mirroring are similar, but mirroring refers to a correspondence between different body parts that have anatomical and developmental similarities. For instance, the hands and feet are mirrors to one another, as are the knees and elbows, and the shoulders and hips. This means we may use points on the hands to treat conditions of the feet, points on the elbows to treat the knees, and points on the shoulders to treat the hips. When using mirroring in clinic it is essential to use corresponding meridian systems. For example, if there is pain around PC 7 on the left arm, we could use LV 4 on the right foot, and ST 41 on the left foot.

For pain located on the left knee, we would mirror the knee to the elbow and select the appropriate points based on the meridian systems. If the pain is located on the LV meridian we could use points located on either the PC or LI channels; remember that the LV connects to the PC through the jue yin, and to the LI through system two. Before moving much further into our discussion we need to cover the importance of contra-lateral needling as it is used in the meridian systems methods.

Contra-Lateral Needling

Contra-lateral needling is defined as needling on the opposite side as the pain, and this method is widespread in meridian based approaches to acupuncture. The most basic technique will needle the same area or point that is expressing symptoms, but on the opposite side of the symptom. For example, carpal tunnel pain located on the right wrist in the region of PC 6 and PC 7, could be treated by needling PC 6 and PC 7 on the left side. Similarly, an acute knee sprain on the left side with pain in the area of GB 34 could be treated with GB 34 on the right side. Although this technique is not widely used, it does have some clinical application in the treatment of acute conditions where one should not needle into the traumatized tissues.

A more common method of contra-lateral needling is to use system one correspondences in places that mirror the affected area. Using the above example of pain on the right wrist at PC 6 and PC 7, we would first mirror the hand to the foot, and then recall that the PC links to the LV in system one. This means we could needle LV points on the left side, in the area of the ankle, and in this case needling LV 3 and LV 4 would be most appropriate. For an acute knee sprain on the left side with pain at ST 35, we would want to needle LI 11 on the right side.

This method of using mirroring and imaging with system one correspondences, and needling on the opposite side of the symptoms, is a foundational technique in various styles of meridian based therapy. It is used extensively in Tung style approaches, in Dr. Tan's methods, and is fundamental to meridian circuit systems as well. The table on the following page shows some common examples of using contra-lateral needling.

Contra-Lateral Needling for Common Conditions

Right Temple Headaches GB channel	Left side: SJ 1, SJ 3, SJ 5
Left Knee Pain at ST 35	Right side: LI 11, LI 4 or LK
Right Knee Pain at LV 7 – LV 8	Left side: PC 3, PC 6
Right Sided Carpal Tunnel Pain at PC 6 and PC 7	Left side: LV 3, LV 4
Left Neck Pain at UB 10 – UB 11	Right side: SI 3, SI 5

In summary, when using system one associations needle on the opposite side of the symptoms, and use appropriate mirroring and imaging techniques. The hands mirror the feet, the elbows mirror the knees, and the hips and shoulders mirror each other as well. In imaging, the hands and feet image the head, and the long bones image the spine and torso. In the above examples SJ 1 and SJ 3 are used for temple headaches because the hand images the head, and the SJ connects to the GB in system one. Similarly, SI 3 and SI 5 may be used for neck pain in the UB channel, the distal end of the metacarpal bone images the neck, and SI 5 images the area where the head connects to the neck. In the example of LI 11 and LK treating pain at ST 35, this is due to the elbow mirroring the knee and the system one connection between the LI and ST meridians.

As a final note contra-lateral needling should be done when using system one, three, and five. This means that for left knee pain at ST 35, we can needle LI 11, SP 9, and SP 10 on the right side. The ST and LI share a system one and five association, and the ST and SP have a system three connection. For left side knee pain on the LV channel we could choose to needle, on the right side, any of the following point combinations: PC 3 and PC 6, or LI 11 and LK, or LU 5 and LU 10.

When meridians are linked through system two or system four, points may be needled contra-laterally or on the same side as the pain. So for the example of pain at ST 35, PC 3 may be needled either contra-laterally or unilaterally. This is because the ST and PC share system two and system four associations. Likewise, left knee pain affecting the LV meridian, can be treated with LI 11 and LK on either the opposite side or the same side. This is because the LI and LV are linked through system two. In cases like this where either side may be needled it is best to palpate the points to find which ones are most reactive and sensitive to pressure.

Selecting the Best Points

The examples above bring up an important point, which is, how to choose the most appropriate and effective points when there are numerous ones to select from. This consideration applies to other systems of acupuncture as well, because for any given condition there are always numerous points indicated. This brings up a fundamental concept in Oriental medicine, that is:

Deciding what points to use is determined by the pattern that is present.

This is the case in traditional forms of acupuncture as well as in meridian based approaches. However, in meridian circuit systems we determine patterns based on the five systems and the patient's top three health priorities. To take the above example of left sided knee pain on the liver meridian, we could needle either PC 3 or LU 5 on the right side. To determine what point would be best, we need to find out what the patient's other health priorities are. If the patient has a secondary concern of insomnia or heart disease it would be best to needle PC 3. In contrast, if the patient suffers from asthma, bronchitis, or some other respiratory condition it would be wise to select LU 5.

Now suppose the same patient had a secondary complaint of a chronic bladder condition. In this case it would be better to needle the lung point, as the LU and UB are connected in system two and four, and LU 5 is the water point on the metal meridian. Therefore, LU 5 would be treating the knee pain on the LV channel, as well as the urinary bladder disease.

This is a brief introduction to how a meridian based approach to pattern identification and treatment allows the doctor to select points that are simultaneously treating numerous symptoms. When this system is mastered it is possible to use 4-8 needles for most treatment sessions. To do this we need to know the five systems, and be able to identify patterns based on the relationships between the meridians. In the next chapter we will cover how to take a meridian based approach to syndrome differentiation.

CHAPTER 4

MERIDIAN CIRCUIT SYSTEMS AND SYNDROME DIFFERENTIATION

There are three steps to determining a meridian based pattern, and when each of these have been mastered, the efficiency and accuracy of the diagnostic process can be greatly increased. Let's now look at each of these steps in detail.

Step 1 - Inquire About the Patient's Top Three Health Concerns.

A key technique in meridian circuit systems is to ask the patient what their top three health priorities are. This has several advantages with the most obvious being that it helps both the client and the doctor to prioritize various symptoms the patient may have. Doing this also helps to determine what patterns are present, and in complex cases where multiple syndromes occur, it helps to identify the ones that are most pertinent.

Another advantage of using this method, is that the doctor is giving space for the patient to express their most pressing needs. This allows the therapist to discover the most problematic symptoms the patient has, and allows the patient to open up in ways that they may not otherwise be able to do so.

Before inquiring too deeply into the primary concern, I find that it is best to briefly ask the patient what their top three health concerns are. This allows the doctor to have a more holistic perspective right from the beginning. When initially discussing each of these concerns with the client, it is appropriate to briefly ask about accompanying symptoms, but it is often best to know what the three chief complaints are before getting into too much detail about any one of them.

Another advantage of doing this is that it helps to prevent any subjective tendencies the therapist may have about arriving at a diagnosis. By allowing the client to express their top three concerns, the doctor is able to be more objective about what symptoms are most problematic for the client. This prevents the therapist from leading the patient during the intake. If the doctor is not careful about this, the very questions they may ask can lead the patient into the doctor's subjective tendencies towards arriving at a diagnosis. This can be avoided by simply allowing the client to express their main concerns.

When the client's needs are prioritized in the way just described, it helps to determine where the most pertinent imbalances are located, and often a pattern can be ascertained just from knowing their top three concerns.

Step 2 - Determine what Meridians are Affected.

The next step when using meridian systems theory is to determine what meridians are symptomatic. For any condition where the symptoms exist on the body, it is essential to determine what meridians are affected. This needs to be done precisely so that meridians are not confused with one another. For instance, when neck pain is a concern it is essential to differentiate between the UB,

GB, SJ, SI, and DU channels. To determine exactly where the symptoms are located palpation should be done very thoroughly. The importance of diagnosing through palpation cannot be over emphasized in this system.

For conditions like pain, stiffness, numbness, and skin conditions, it is easy to determine the affected meridians through palpation or observation. However, for conditions like constipation, fatigue, or anxiety, there is often no location on the body where symptoms exist.

For symptoms or diseases that are not localized on the body, determine what meridians or organs are most likely to be involved by using established Chinese medical knowledge. This can be done by using zang-fu methods, observing the tongue and pulse, doing a differential diagnosis, or by asking about accompanying symptoms. When questioning, be careful not to lead the patient through the questions. Alternately, ask the patient about their other concerns, as this will often help to identify what pattern is present.

Step 3 - Use the 5 Systems to Determine a Meridian Based Pattern.

When analyzing the patient's chief concerns and affected meridians, we need to arrive at an understanding of what meridians are most out of balance, and which ones would respond best to treatment. To do this requires us to account for their top three health priorities, while using the five systems to develop what I call a 4 meridian (4M) circuit.

A 4M circuit is defined as four meridians that are interconnected through the five systems.

43

Let's now examine the concept and process of arriving at a diagnosis based on the method of using 4M circuits.

After the first two steps have been completed your notes should have sequentially listed the client's top three concerns, and the most likely affected meridians and organs. Listed below is an example from an actual case study.

Male, 48

Primary Concern – Frequent, urgent, painful urination, UB

Secondary Concern – Impotence, KI

Third Concern – Constipation, LI

The patient had suffered from urgent and painful urination for over two years, and Western medical tests were inconclusive as to the cause. The pain was located right at the tip of the urethra, and an urgent bearing down sensation was present in the region of the bladder organ. Although the bearing down sensation transversed through the RN, KI, and ST meridians, the condition obviously involved the bladder, and for that reason it was the organ that was listed as being affected. The secondary complaint of impotence is related to the kidney function in Chinese medicine, and the third concern of constipation involves the large intestine.

From the beginning it is obvious that there is an association between the UB and KI as they relate to the primary and secondary concerns. We can represent this connection as such:

UB - KI

The next step, and this is the crucial one in determining patterns based on a meridian systems perspective, is to identify a 4M circuit. Remember that the 4M circuit is defined as four meridians that are connected to one another through the five meridian systems.

To create a 4M circuit, we take two pairs that connect to another pair, through the five systems. In the above example, we find that the LI is the organ involved in the patient's tertiary concern, and we also know that the LI connects to the KI in system four, thus we can add the LI.

UB - KI

-

LI

Our next task to complete a 4M circuit is to find which meridian connects to both the LI and UB. To determine this we simply look at the connections for the LI and UB, and find a meridian that is shared between them. The meridian associations for the LI and UB are as follows:

LI - ST - LV - <u>LU</u> - KI - ST

UB - SI - <u>LU</u> - KI - <u>LU</u> - SI

When we compare the LI and UB connections we find that the LU links to both of them. We can now add the LU to complete the circuit.

UB - KI

-     -

LU - LI

Interesting enough, when I asked the patient if he had a fourth concern, he told me he has suffered from asthma since being a kid.

The above example demonstrates how a meridian systems approach can often predict and determine where other health problems are. In addition, I have also found that it is very effective for revealing root patterns of imbalance. Let's look at another case study to see how a meridian systems approach can do this.

Female, 54

Primary Concern – Left side knee pain along the liver channel, LV

Secondary Concern – Left side sinus congestion, LI and ST

Tertiary Concern – Headaches behind the eyes, LV; Hot flashes from menopause, KI

The tongue was large, red, dry, with cracks in the ST, LV, and KI regions. It alternated between having a thick yellow coat and no coat at all.

The location of the knee pain was easy to assess, it started near LV 7 and ran up to LV 8. Palpation revealed that these points were very reactive. The sinus congestion was worse on the left side in the region of LI 20 and occasionally she felt it near ST 3. The congestion was induced by allergies. Her third concern of headaches were located behind the eyes, and they frequently occurred with photosensitivity; for this reason they were listed as a LV pattern headache. The hot flashes were a menopausal symptom and are therefore listed as a KI pattern.

In this patient the chief complaint is liver channel knee pain, and the secondary concern is sinus congestion mostly around the LI meridian. In system two the LI and LV are connected, therefore, we can take this pair as being the primary meridians to work with. When I recognize a primary pair I will write it in my notes as such:

LI - LV

To treat the left sided knee pain we may needle LI 11 and LI 4 on the right or left side. This utilizes the technique of mirroring the knee to the elbow, LI 4 is added for its ability to resolve pain.

Also notice how needling LI 4 helps to resolve the second complaint of sinus congestion, and even the third concern of headaches behind the eyes. This example demonstrates how meridian systems theory can effectively treat many conditions simultaneously with fewer needles.

Let's now contrast this with a zang-fu approach. Typically zang-fu methods would approach knee pain as being related to a kidney deficiency, there may be other reasons such as cold, damp, injury, or surgery, but it is very common to think of knee conditions as being related to the kidneys. With the patient's age, and frequent occurrence of hot flashes, it would be easy to conclude that a kidney deficiency was present, and it was, she was right in the middle of menopause.

If the doctor were to use zang-fu methods they would probably start asking about other kidney related symptoms like lumbar pain, night sweats, etc. Many of these symptoms were also present, *but* they were not the client's main concerns. A traditional approach to treating the knee pain could have easily arrived at the diagnosis of a kidney yin deficiency, and then developed a corresponding treatment based on that alone. This may have even been done without questioning the patient about *h e r* other health concerns.

If the doctor was wise enough to ask her about her other priorities, and he is using a zang-fu approach, then things get really complicated. The knee pain was on the liver meridian, and there is also the presence of liver pattern headaches. The apparent kidney yin deficiency signs could be connected to the liver symptoms, and it would be possible to arrive at the diagnosis of a liver-kidney yin deficiency. This is fine, but what about the secondary concern of sinus congestion which is related to allergies? If we follow this pattern through we find that the patient suffered from allergies to pollens and food. When severe the lungs would get congested and she would suffer from shortness of breath. The food allergies would frequently cause bloating, water retention, and diarrhea. From these symptoms it was apparent that spleen and lung patterns were present, and they were compounded with excess damp-phlegm accumulation; this is why the tongue sometimes had a thick coat.

We now have ourselves in the middle of a complex pattern: liver and kidney yin deficiency, with spleen and lung qi patterns, and damp-phlegm accumulation. All of this was compounded with countless symptoms for each organ.

Where is one to start developing a treatment strategy for a client like this?

**We start by asking the patient what
their top three health concerns are.**

Let's return to the meridian systems approach. We left off identifying the LI and LV meridians as being the primary pair to work with, and remember we found that LI 11 and LI 4 could simultaneously treat the knee pain, sinus congestion, and headaches, and we only have to needle one side. While this two point combination can treat the top concerns, it does not address the underlying patterns;

48

however, this is where we start to use meridian circuit systems to determine the best approach for treating the root conditions. To do this we need to understand the final step in developing treatments based on the meridian circuit systems.

In regards to our current case study we found that the LI and LV were the most obvious pair to work with; however, we also want to address the root patterns of disharmony. To do this we need to identify a 4M circuit. Remember that a 4M circuit is composed of two meridian pairs that connect to one another through the five systems. To determine what circuit is most out of balance in our current case study, let's review the meridian connections for the LI and LV. These connections are:

LI - ST - LV - LU - KI - ST

LV - PC - LI - GB - SI - LU

Starting with our initial pair of the LI and LV, we want to find one meridian that connects to the LI, one meridian that connects to the LV, and each of these new meridians must also connect to each other.

Since the patient also complained of hot flashes, and has many other signs and symptoms of kidney deficiency, let's form a connection between the LI and KI. This leaves us with the following:

LI - LV

-

KI

Now we need to find a meridian that connects to both the KI and LV, and reviewing the associations between them we find that the PC links with both of them.

49

This leaves us with the following 4M circuit:

LI - LV

-   -

KI - PC

These then represent the meridians we will use to treat the patient. We have already determined that the LI 4, LI 11 combination will address the left sided knee pain, sinus congestion, and liver related headaches. We should also needle LV points, so let's select LV 3 on the left side for this patient, as well as KI 3 and KI 9.

The PC's role in this circuit is very powerful, as PC 3 and PC 6 can treat the knee pain in the LV channel. Similarly, PC 6 has a variety of functions that assist in the overall pattern, it resolves liver qi stagnation, moves phlegm, opens the Yin Wei, and benefits the yin. Amazing enough, the pericardium's diverse functions are able to address the complex zang-fu patterns that the patient had.

This example demonstrates the ease with which a meridian systems approach allows for identifying root and branch patterns, and leads to determining effective treatment strategies. When meridian systems theory is combined with prioritizing the patient's top concerns, it provides a clear structure for identifying the most pertinent patterns of disharmony. In the next chapter we will begin to discuss some of the 4M circuits that can be created from the meridian systems correspondences.

CHAPTER 5

THE 4 MERIDIAN CIRCUITS

This chapter will build on the concepts of the five meridian systems and the theory of 4M circuits. These are essential ideas to understand when using a meridian based approach to pattern identification in the treatment of internal conditions. To begin, lets look at the first four channels in the sequential flow of qi through the 12 regular meridians.

The LU is considered to be the first meridian and its time is from 3 a.m. to 5 a.m. After this the qi moves into the LI meridian and then to the ST. In regards to the connection between the LU and LI we refer to this as an internal-external relationship, or a system three connection. The association between the LI and ST is a system one correspondence, and this may also be referred to as the yang ming pair. After the qi exits the ST meridian it moves to the SP, and the ST and SP are linked in system three as an internal-external pair.

With close examination we find that the LU and SP are connected through the tai yin pairing, or what we may also refer to as a system one correspondence.

Taking the relationship between these four meridians we can create the following 4M circuit.

LU - LI
-　　-
SP - ST

This same type of rational can also be applied to the other channels as we follow the flow of qi through the circuit of the 12 regular meridians. When done we find the following 4M circuits emerge.

HT - SI　　　　　　　　　　　　　PC - SJ
-　　-　　　　and　　　　-　　-
KI - UB　　　　　　　　　　　　　LV - GB

Connecting four meridians according to the five meridian systems allows us to form the above circuits and various others. We shall now cover all the possible 4M circuits that may be formed, as well as the functions and indications of each of these. To begin we will start by reviewing the tai yang and examining the pairs that can connect to it.

TAI YANG (SI – UB)

Areas Influenced: Eyes, head, neck, shoulders, back, and spine. The most posterior portions of the yang aspect of the arms, back, and legs.

Functions:

1) Circulates qi through the tai yang.

2) Opens the DU mai.

3) Distributes wei qi to the surface of the body and regulates the immune system.

4) Regulates fluids through the functions of the small intestine and bladder.

The tai yang connects to three other meridian pairs: the tai yin, the shao yin, and the lung and liver. These circuits may be represented as follows.

UB - SI	UB - SI	UB - SI
- -	- -	- -
LU - SP	KI - HT	LU - LV

When tai yang conditions occur with secondary or tertiary complaints in the lungs or spleen, use the tai yang-tai yin circuit. When the primary complaint involves the tai yang, and the secondary or tertiary concerns point to either the heart or kidneys, it is best to use the tai yang-shao yin circuit. If liver or lungs patterns present with symptoms in the tai yang, use the tai yang-lung/liver circuit. Let's now examine each of these circuits in greater detail.

The Tai Yang – Tai Yin Circuit

$$UB - SI$$
$$- \quad -$$
$$LU - SP$$

Functions:

1) Regulates the Tai Yang and Tai Yin.

2) Benefits Wei Qi.

3) Governs Qi (Lungs govern qi, spleen governs post-natal qi).

4) Controls Fluid and Water Metabolism.

Primary Concerns: Occipital headaches, pain within the neck, shoulders, back, and spine, eye diseases, urinary conditions.

2nd or 3rd Concerns: Fatigue, respiratory and digestive symptoms, allergies, low appetite, bloating, diarrhea, low immune function, edema, sadness, and depression.

Explanation:

This circuit is to be used when the primary symptoms exist within the tai yang. This includes conditions of the neck, back, shoulders, and spine as well as diseases of the immune system and bladder. This circuit is used when secondary symptoms involving the tai yin are also present. These include conditions such as bronchitis, weak immunity, poor digestion, water retention, or other symptoms that clearly involve the tai yin organs or meridians.   Primary symptoms affecting the tai yang channels that also occur with qi deficiency of the lungs and spleen are to be treated with this circuit.

Neck and Back Pain – The Most Common Tai Yang Symptoms

The most common symptoms affecting the tai yang meridians are neck, back, shoulder, lumbar pain, sciatica, and neuralgia along the SI and UB channels. When pain is present along the UB meridian SI points may be needled for good therapeutic effects. Most notably are the points SI 3, SI 4, SI 5, and SI 6.   Using the imaging methods of relating long bones to the spine, we find that SI 3 and SI 5 are most appropriate for neck pain, SI 4 for lumbar pain, and SI 6 for scapular and upper back pain.   In Tung's points we find that 22.08 and 22.09, located between SI 3 and SI 4, are indicated for sciatica, back pain, and pain at the popliteal fossa, this is explained by the connection between the hand and foot tai yang meridians.

Points on the UB Meridian to Treat Lung Related Conditions

The Tung acupuncture points of Qi Hu (77.26) are a three-point unit.   The first point is located 1.5 cun posterior to the lateral malleolus, the second point is 2 cun above the first, and the third point is located 2 cun above the second point. These points are indicated for pain in the shoulder, clavicle, and scapula, as well as costal pain due to pleurisy. When used for shoulder pain the points are best utilized when the pain is located along either the LU or SI meridian.   Its ability to treat scapular pain is due to its system one connection with the SI, while the indication for pleurisy is from its system two association with the LU.

The Small Intestine and Spleen Connection

In addition to treating neck pain SI 5 is a fire point on a fire meridian, it is therefore useful for treating spleen deficiency. This point is effectively employed when the patient's main complaint is neck pain, and they also present with a secondary concern associated with spleen deficiency. When this pattern occurs it is also helpful to use SP 3, as a little known indication of SP 3 is that it strengthens the spine. This can be understood due to the spleen's connection to the tai yang, as well as its location at the distal portion of a long bone. This is similar to the function and location of SI 3, as they are reverse mirrors of each other. SP 3 is appropriate to use when there is spinal pain with spleen deficiency.

The Lung Meridian in the Treatment of Bladder Diseases

Many conditions involving the urinary bladder organ are also treated with this circuit. Since the lungs and spleen are primary organs involved in water metabolism, points on the tai yin are useful for conditions such as incontinence and urinary infections. The primary points on the lung channel for bladder conditions are LU 5 and LU 7. This point combination is especially useful because it synergizes numerous styles of acupuncture therapy. In meridian systems theory the LU and UB are paired through system two and four. Lung 5 is located at the elbow, which images the navel, and the navel is in close proximity to the anatomical location of the urinary bladder. In 5-element theory, LU 5 is the water point on a metal meridian, and therefore has a strong influence on water energies. The effect LU 7 has on bladder diseases is due to it being the opening point for the RN mai, which passes right through the area of the bladder.

56

An example of when to use the tai yang-tai yin circuit would be a client whose primary concern is mid-thoracic pain along the UB meridian, suffers from a secondary concern of asthma, and has a tertiary complaint of frequently catching colds. While traditional zang-fu approaches would most likely identify a lung and spleen pattern, meridian systems theory would identify an imbalance in the tai yang-tai yin circuit.

THE TAI YANG – SHAO YIN CIRCUIT

UB - SI
- -
KI - HT

Functions:

1) Regulates the Tai Yang and Shao Yin.

2) Governs Blood and Essence.

3) Regulates Fluid Metabolism.

Primary Concerns: Neck, back, shoulder, and lumbar pain, occipital headaches, eye diseases, urinary conditions, pain or symptoms in the tai yang channels.

2nd or 3rd Concerns: Palpitations, heart disease, anemia, poor memory, tinnitus, osteoporosis, infertility, impotence, amenorrhea, menopause.

Explanation:

The tai yang connects to the qi and yang aspects of the nervous system, while the shao yin links to the nervous system through the blood, essence, marrow, and spirit. Whenever imbalance is present in the tai yang the condition of the heart, blood, kidneys, and essence should be assessed. Clearly differentiating between tai yang conditions of the qi level (LU – SP), and the blood/essence level (HT – KI), is key to getting long-term results and treating root patterns. When the heart and kidneys are contributing to symptoms within the tai yang the patient will express typical shao yin symptoms such as palpitations, poor memory, anxiety, dizziness, low back pain, shen disturbance, bone disorders, and reproductive or urinary symptoms. Blood and essence deficiencies are also common.

The Heart

It is common for various heart patterns to influence the tai yang channels since they have a shared connection. While the tai yang is associated with the DU, the heart correlates with the spirit and the conscious aspects of being. When imbalances and pain exist in the tai yang channels it is imperative to determine if the heart plays a role in the etiology of the disease. This may occur if there is a deficiency of heart blood or yin. Likewise, shen disturbance that is based in a heart imbalance may affect the tai yang and cause a variety of symptoms or diseases. Since both the blood and shen strongly affect nervous system functions, it is important to be able to identify when heart imbalances are contributing to symptoms within the tai yang.

The Kidneys

Kidney deficiency frequently affects the tai yang meridians and can lead to symptoms in the eyes, ears, head, neck, shoulders, back, and spine. The kidneys are vital to the tai yang because they store and transform the essence, and the transmutation from essence to marrow is essential to proper nervous system functioning. Whenever the tai yang channels are diseased a differential diagnosis should be applied to determine if the kidneys are the primary yin organ underlying the symptoms or not.

Luo Connecting Point, HT 5

Some sources indicate that one of the functions of HT 5 is to benefit the bladder. This has been explained because the heart and the small intestine are internally/externally related, and the SI and UB form the tai yang pair. Similarly, the HT and KI are connected through system one, so the heart luo point can also benefit the bladder by way of its connection to the kidney. This can also be understood when the forearm is imaged to the lumbar-sacral area, and the hands are imaged to the genitals. Both imaging and systems theory explains why HT 5 may be used for urinary conditions.

The Heart Meridian in the Treatment of Neck and Shoulder Pain

Since the heart meridian connects to the SI and GB channels it can be useful for treating neck and shoulder pain. Using heart points to treat these areas is most appropriate when the patient also presents with heart signs and symptoms. For neck and shoulder pain in the SI or GB meridians, palpate the area of HT 4 – HT 7 feeling for areas of tightness or reactivity.

The Wrist and Ankles Image the Neck and Throat, KI 6 and LU 7

There are many examples in traditional point indications that correlate with the theory of imaging the wrist and ankles to the neck and throat. Notably, KI 6 opens the Yin Qiao, which passes through the throat and has crossing points with ST 9 and ST 12. In addition, LU 7 is coupled to KI 6 and is useful for easing sore throats and treating neck pain.

Imaging the Ankle to the Neck and Shoulder, UB 62

In imaging the ankle to the neck we find that UB 62 is the beginning and opening point for the Yang Qiao, and the Yang Qiao terminates at GB 20. In reverse imaging, the ankle may be used to treat the shoulder, and we find that the Yang Qiao has crossing points at SI 10, SJ 15, LI 15, and LI 16. These two examples are a demonstration of how the 8 extra-ordinary meridians overlap with the theory of imaging.

TAI YANG – QI DISPERSION CICUIT

SI - UB
- -
LV - LU

Functions:

1) Regulates the Tai Yang, Liver, and Lungs.

2) Disperses Qi (LU) and Promotes the Smooth Flow of Qi (LV).

3) Benefits Wei Qi.

Primary Concerns: Head, eyes, neck, shoulder, back and spinal conditions that involve the tai yang channels, conditions involving the bladder or small intestine.

2nd or 3rd Concerns: LU or LV imbalances, cough, chest tightness, impaired immunity, allergies, liver diseases.

Explanation:

This circuit plays a major role in the circulation and dispersion of qi through the entire body. While the tai yang circulates qi through their respective pathways, the lungs function to disperse qi, and the liver promotes the smooth flow of qi. This makes this circuit essential for conditions of qi stagnation when the spine, back, shoulders, and tai yang channels are involved.

Since the liver governs the smooth flow of qi through the entire body, liver qi stagnation can easily influence the neck and shoulders. This may occur in the GB meridian, as well as the SI meridian, since the SI and LV are connected through system four. For this reason liver stagnation can easily effect the neck, back, scapula, and shoulders. Primary liver points for relieving pain in the SI meridian in these areas are LV 3, LV 4, and LV 5.

Similar to the liver's function of governing the smooth flow of qi, is the lungs role in governing and dispersing the qi. When the lungs are functioning properly the metal energy balances the wood energy of the liver. However, if the functions of the lungs are compromised, the qi of the liver may stagnate and overact on other organs. In this circuit the liver will overact on either the small intestine or lungs, and cause characteristic symptoms such as shoulder tension, coughing, and chest tightness.

Since the tai yang meridians may combine with the tai yin meridians, as well as with the LV and LU, it is especially important to distinguish which of the yin organs is most out of balance. When the primary symptoms exist within the tai yang, and there are also lung signs present, be sure to differentiate between a greater imbalance in the liver or spleen.

SI 7, The Luo-Connecting Point

Like many luo-connecting points SI 7 connects to more than just its internally/externally related meridian. In addition to connecting to the heart, SI 7 also connects to the liver and urinary bladder meridians. It is known to be a point for treating liver related emotional patterns, and it works with UB 58 to supplement the yang for mental clarity.

SI 3, The Du Mai and Liver Patterns

The point SI 3 can be very useful for treating a number of liver patterns that manifest with symptoms in the head, neck, spine, and nervous system. Traditionally, SI 3 is indicated for internal wind, and this is usually explained because of it being the opening point for the DU. However, if we review the pattern of internal wind we find that it is due to liver yang rising; so another way to understand the ability of SI 3 to address internal wind is due to the small intestines association with the liver.

Summary

The tai yang-LV/LU circuit is a commonly used circuit that is appropriate for upper back pain due to qi stagnation. It is to be used when the primary concern involves the tai yang, and liver or lungs imbalances are also present.

YANG MING (LI – ST)

Areas Influenced: Face and sinuses, stomach, abdomen, and intestines. The yang ming meridians transverse the most anterior regions of the yang portions of the body.

Functions

1) Regulates Digestion.

2) Harmonizes Intestines.

3) Controls Bowel Functions.

The yang ming combines with three other meridian pairs to form circuits that primarily treat digestive and bowel conditions. Whenever the client's main concern involves the stomach or bowels, the yang ming should be considered as a pair. To determine root patterns and account for secondary symptoms it is essential to identify which yin organs are also involved in the disease pathogenesis. The yang ming pairs with the tai yin, the jue yin, and the PC and KI. These three circuits are represented below.

ST - LI	ST - LI	ST - LI
- -	- -	- -
SP - LU	PC - LV	PC - KI

When lung and spleen symptoms present with a primary concern involving the yang ming, work with the yang ming -tai yin circuit. For yang ming patterns that clearly present with liver imbalances use the yang ming - jue yin circuit. This circuit is also very beneficial when stress or emotional disharmony contributes to the overall pattern.

65

The yang ming also pairs with the KI and PC meridians, and this circuit is useful for yang ming patterns that occur with kidney deficiencies, or disharmony in the Yin Qiao and Yin Wei meridians. Let's now examine each of these three circuits in greater detail.

YANG MING – TAI YIN CIRCUIT

ST - LI

\- -

SP - LU

Functions:

1) Regulates Digestion, Intestine, and Bowel Functions.

2) Governs Qi through Respiration and Digestion.

3) Regulates Water Metabolism.

Primary Complaints: Constipation, diarrhea, diabetes, sinusitis, rhinitis, stomach ulcers, gastritis, colitis, etc.

2nd and 3rd Concerns: Food allergies, fatigue, low appetite, bloating, edema, asthma, bronchitis, various lung and digestive conditions.

Explanation:

The yang ming is connected to the tai yin through their internal-external relationship, and for this reason conditions that involve the yang ming frequently occur with pathologies in the tai yin. When the yang ming are in a state of imbalance it is always important to determine if the tai yin are also involved or are contributing to the pattern. Since the yang organs are prone to excess, and the yin to deficiency, it is often the case that the yang ming will manifest excessive patterns while the tai yin manifests deficiencies. Patterns of qi deficiency in the lungs or spleen occurring with primary symptoms in the yang ming are treated using this circuit. This may include conditions such as diarrhea, constipation, poor digestion, allergies, and sinus congestion.

Respiratory disorders that are influenced by the digestion are usually treated with this circuit. This includes conditions like Candida and food allergies. For these types of disorders it is common for phlegm to occur in the lungs as a result of root imbalances in the digestive system. This is conveyed through the traditional saying of "the spleen is the producer of phlegm and the lungs are the container of phlegm."

Stomach Points for Lung Conditions:

It is well known that ST 40 is indicated for resolving phlegm in the lungs, and ST 36 is beneficial for strengthening the lungs. In Master Tung's system there are also numerous points on the stomach channel that are useful for lung disorders. Noteworthy, are Master Tung's points 77.08, 77.09, and 77.10; these points are located near ST 36, ST 38, and ST 39, and are indicated for asthma. The point 77.09 also treats TB, pulmonary edema, emphysema, and lung tumors. Similarly, the points 88.17, 88.18, and 88.19 are located on the thigh of the ST channel, they are indicated for lung diseases and dermatological conditions.

The above example of ST points treating lung syndromes illustrates a common pattern we will observe when working with 4M circuits; which is, meridians within a 4M circuit have a strong effect on each other. So even though the LU and ST are not directly connected, they can influence each other because of their shared relationships with the SP and LI.

YANG MING – JUE YIN CIRCUIT

ST - LI

-　　-

PC - LV

Functions:

1) Regulates Digestive and Bowel Functions.

2) Calms the Shen.

3) Harmonizes Digestion through Regulating Qi and Blood Circulation.

Primary Complaints: Stress induced digestive and abdominal conditions, constipation, IBS, loss of appetite, ulcers, colitis.

2nd and 3rd Concerns: Irritability, anger, stress, chest tightness, palpitations, heart disease, headaches, plum pit syndrome, PMS.

Explanation:

This circuit should be used whenever the primary symptoms exist within the yang ming and occur with liver, pericardium, or qi and blood stagnation symptoms. Proper circulation of the qi and blood is essential to good digestive health, and when liver patterns present they can easily influence the stomach and large intestine. This can cause symptoms such as acid reflux, ulcers, stomach pain, constipation, and IBS. When the liver is involved in yang ming patterns it is common that the client will also suffer from excessive stress, frustration, and anger. For these reasons PC points are an important addition to the treatment since they have the functions of moving liver qi, calming the mind, and harmonizing the stomach and intestines.

Pericardium 3 and PC 6 are an especially useful combination for yang ming conditions that occur with liver patterns

> "The luo of the stomach travels up to the heart,"
>
> *Chapter 49, Nei Jing*

and shen disturbance. In terms of 8 principles and 5 elements, the pericardium is between wood and fire, and can reduce wood excesses while supplementing earth deficiencies. It can also reduce or supplement the fire element depending on needle technique and point combinations. Therefore, PC 3 and PC 6 is a very powerful point combination that appears in several circuits that involve the digestive system. This point combination is irreplaceable in most digestive patterns.

The Stomach, Abdomen, and Pericardium Meridian

In meridian systems theory the pericardium connects to most of the major meridians flowing through the abdomen. The pericardium has a system one association with the liver, a system two connection to the stomach, and links with the kidney through system five. It also shares association with the spleen through the coupling of SP 4 and PC 6, and

ST

LV   PC   SP

KI

the Yin Wei crosses with KI 9, SP 13, SP 15, and SP 16. These relationships make the pericardium meridian especially effective for a variety of abdominal and chest conditions. Due to the pericardium's strong association with the abdomen, and its system one connection with the liver, it should be used whenever liver imbalances cause abdominal, digestive, and yang ming patterns.

Master Tung's Points

The points 11.01, 11.02, and 11.05 are located on the index finger and are therefore closely connected to the large intestine meridian. They are indicated for heart disease, palpitations, and hernia. Though the association between heart conditions and hernias are not readily apparent, it can be understood in terms of the jue yin meridians. While liver imbalances are often associated with hernias, palpitations connect to the pericardium. Through the large intestines association with the liver and jue yin, the numerous functions of these points can easily be understood.

Summary

This circuit is very commonly used when digestive and yang ming patterns present with qi and blood stagnation. It is also very useful for abdominal complaints that are caused by stress and shen disturbance.

YANG MING – WATER AND FIRE CIRCUIT

ST - LI
-     -
PC - KI

Functions:

1) Regulates Digestive and Bowel Functions.

2) Influences the Chest and Abdomen.

3) Harmonizes Water and Fire Balance.

4) Supplements Yin.

Primary Complaints: Abdominal pain, constipation, diarrhea, nausea, vomiting, and yang ming patterns.

2ⁿᵈ or 3ʳᵈ Concerns: Tightness in the chest, palpitations, infertility, low back pain, anxiety, kidney or heart disease.

Explanation:

This circuit treats yang ming digestive patterns that occur with kidney and pericardium signs and symptoms. In traditional theory we find that KI 6 regulates the large intestine through its ability to treat constipation, and PC 6 harmonizes the stomach. The pericardium's effect on stomach functions is most well known through the functions of PC 6, and when this point is paired with PC 3 it treats a wide variety of stomach conditions. Since it is a fire meridian it may be used to either clear excessive heat from the stomach, or boost stomach and spleen functions by way of the 5-element cycle. Yang ming patterns that occur with excessive stress, anxiety, or shen disturbance, may also be treated with this circuit, when kidney signs are also present. This may present as an underlying yin deficiency, and the patient may have symptoms such as low back pain, night sweats, five palm sweating, thirst, constipation, or low sex drive.

The Yang Ming, Fire, and Kidney Water Balance

This circuit works wonders for someone with a yang ming pattern that has exhausted their kidney essence and has heat signs in the heart and pericardium. When the kidney essence and yin has been depleted it can cause imbalance by allowing the fire to be in excess. This is common for older men that suffer from heart disease and constipation, and have over-worked and stressed their systems for many years. Menopausal and post-menopausal women also exhibit this pattern when their kidney yin declines and they suffer from heat signs with anxiety, shen disturbance, and constipation. This circuit is appropriate for clients with concurrent symptoms of constipation, heart disease, and kidney deficiency.

The 8 – Extraordinary and Systems Theory, KI 6 and the Yin Qiao

Examining the functions, areas of influence, and coupling points of the extraordinary meridians, reveals numerous examples of the five meridian systems and 4M circuits. The opening point for the Yin Qiao meridian is KI 6, which is a commonly indicated point for constipation. In addition, the Yin Qiao is indicated for abdominal distress due to stagnation of qi and blood, and it has crossing points with ST 9 and ST 12. These correspondences reveal the connections between the kidneys, large intestine, and yang ming pair. Additionally, the ankle images the neck and throat, and ST 9 and ST 12 are both located in the area of the throat.

System Five: KI 6 and PC 6 in Combination

The points KI 6 and PC 6 may be combined for a good effect when yang ming symptoms occur with pericardium and kidney patterns. These points may be used together for a wide variety of stomach, abdominal, and intestinal disorders, when the water and fire balance of the kidneys and pericardium are causative factors. If we examine the functions of the Yin Qiao and Yin Wei we find that both of them influence the chest and abdomen, nourish yin, and connect to the stomach and intestines. In the case of constipation, KI 6 is an empirical point that works best for patterns of yin or blood deficiency. This is due to its ability to supplement the yin, its system four connection with the large intestine, and its influence on the Yin Qiao as it passes through the abdomen.

Although PC points are not typically recommended for constipation, its position in this circuit can be useful for moving qi and blood, descending stomach qi, and clearing heat, all of which can be a helpful adjunct for treating constipation.

The three major zang-fu patterns for constipation are excessive heat, yin deficiency, and qi stagnation. Since the pericardium meridian may be used to clear heat, supplement yin, and move liver qi, it makes this meridian a good addition to conventional points for constipation. This is especially true when palpitations, shen disturbance, or other pericardium symptoms are present.

74

SJ 6, An Empirical Point for Constipation

Often it will be necessary to add an extra meridian to the circuits to get the most well rounded treatment. For instance, let's suppose we have a client with a primary concern of constipation, a secondary concern of low back pain, a history of heart disease, and excessive heat signs. In a case like this we may want to add a point like SJ 6 to treat the constipation and clear the excessive heat. Let's see how the SJ fits into our current circuit.

LI - ST

-   -

KI - PC

-   -

SJ

Notice how the SJ connects to both the KI and PC, and it helps to clear heat while treating constipation. This is a natural addition to our primary circuit, and it brings up a crucial strategy when working with 4M circuits. Learning to add a meridian, or a meridian pair, to a 4M circuit may be necessary to treat the patient's overall pattern. So while it is most beneficial to determine the primary 4M circuit that is expressing disharmony, it is also important to be able to make the proper additions when necessary. Let's look at another example of adding a meridian to our current circuit.

Suppose we have a patient with a primary concern of morning diarrhea, a secondary concern of low back pain, a tertiary complaint of nausea, and a history of heart disease. The patient also frequently feels cold and has a pale puffy tongue. According to zang-fu differentiation the patient has a spleen and kidney yang deficiency. However, since we are using circuit theory to develop our treatment strategy, we decide to use the yang ming – KI/PC circuit, since this circuit can best account for the client's chief concerns. Now while traditional sources say to use kidney, spleen, and stomach points for a spleen and kidney yang deficiency, we want to examine what circuit theory can offer. The first thing we notice is that the LI and PC meridians are part of this circuit, but they are not typically called for in zang-fu point prescriptions when a spleen and kidney yang deficiency pattern exists. However, for a pattern like this the use of LI points should not be overlooked, since LI 10 has similar functions as ST 36, and Ling Ku is able to treat lumbar pain while warming and activating the yang.

In regards to the pericardium's position in this circuit it should be remembered that PC 6 opens the Yin Wei, and the Yin Wei has crossing points with SP 13, SP 15, and SP 16. The pairing of PC 6 and SP 4 is also relevant in that one of the functions of the Chong mai is to connect the pre and post natal qi, and for this reason can be used for conditions of spleen deficiency with a root imbalance in the kidneys. Knowing that PC 6 eases nausea (the client's third concern), and it connects to the above mentioned SP points, we decided to use it in combination with SP 4 so as to open both the Yin Wei and Chong.

When we add the SP meridian to this circuit we find that it connects to the stomach.

LI - ST - SP
-       -
KI - PC

Continuing with this line of thought we may want to supplement yang and fire with the use of the SJ, which incidentally shares functions with the Yin Wei of connecting the pre and post-natal qi between the spleen and kidneys.

The SJ can now be added to the circuit.

$$\text{LI - ST - SP}$$
$$|\quad|\quad|$$
$$\text{KI - PC - SJ}$$

Notice how we started with a pattern of spleen and kidney yang deficiency, and we chose to work with the yang ming - kidney/pericardium circuit based on the client's top three health concerns. Had we went with a traditional zang-fu pattern approach we would have primarily used spleen, stomach, and kidney points; however, with a circuit based approach the addition of the LI, and two fire meridians, give us an unique edge that encompasses 5-element wisdom as well. The fire of the PC and SJ can help to boost the earth energies, while also allowing us to work with the extraordinary vessels.

As a final statement about the functions of this circuit, Ling Ku and Da Bai are both located on the LI meridian, and when combined they are powerful for treating the patient's secondary concern of low back pain. They also supplement, warm, and activate the yang and are therefore very useful for the patient's underlying zang-fu pattern.

Summary

Use this circuit when digestive and bowel conditions occur with kidney deficiency, back pain, and shen disturbance. It may also be used for patterns where the fire and water balance of the digestive organs are disturbed.

SHAO-YANG (SJ - GB)

Areas Influenced: Head, neck, shoulders, costal regions, and hips. The shao yang meridians also have a major influence on the mind, emotions, and neurological system.

FUNCTIONS:

1) Distributes Qi through the Shao Yang Channels.

2) Influences the Mind and Emotions.

3) Resolves Wind.

The connection between the shao yang and conditions of the mind and emotions are extremely important but not frequently spoken of in traditional theory. We can most easily understand this by way that the shao yang connects to both the jue yin and the shao yin. The GB connects to both the HT and LV, while the SJ connects to the PC and KI. It is through these associations with the yin organs that the shao yang becomes a major meridian pair for influencing mental and emotional conditions. In addition, since both shao yang meridians pass through the head, neck, and shoulders, they have an intensive association with the nervous system. This can be seen in the way in which they are used to treat conditions such as strokes, epilepsy, Parkinson's, and other major conditions that affect the neurological system.

Besides connecting to the jue yin and shao yin, the shao yang pair also connects with the spleen and heart. The three circuits of the shao yang are represented on the next page.

```
GB  -  SJ          GB  -  SJ          GB  -  SJ
-      -           -      -           -      -
LV  -  PC          HT  -  KI          HT  -  SP
```

Let's now take a closer look at each of these circuits in greater detail.

SHAO YANG – JUE YIN CIRCUIT

GB - SJ
-   -
LV - PC

Functions:

1) Circulates Qi through the Shao Yang and Jue Yin.

2) Calms the Shen.

3) Controls Circulation of Qi and Blood.

4) Resolves Wind.

Primary Concerns: Temple headaches, neck pain, insomnia, seizures, strokes, anxiety, hyperthyroidism, epilepsy, hip pain, Parkinson's, shen disturbance, tightness in the ribs, constipation.

2nd or 3rd Concerns: Chest tightness, costal pain, stress, PMS, irritability, abdominal pain, palpitations, groin pain.

Explanation:

This circuit is often used for conditions of the head, neck, throat, shoulders and hips, when the shao yang meridians are in a state of disharmony. Shao yang symptoms will often occur with jue yin patterns due to the internal-external relationship they share. It is often the case that liver patterns will influence the GB meridian and present with symptoms such as temple headaches, neck tension, eye disorders, and insomnia.

This circuit is also very powerful for clearing internal heat and fire that is located in the shao yang and jue yin meridians. Liver fire will often manifest with GB meridian symptoms, and the SJ is effective for relieving symptoms associated with both the gallbladder and liver. When liver fire is present, needling the SJ helps to clear fire, while the PC meridian clears heat and resolves liver stagnation.

The San Jiao and Gallbladder

It is widely known that points on the SJ meridian, especially SJ 5, may be used to treat liver patterns such as liver yang rising and liver fire. San jiao 5 is commonly used for temple headaches, and this reveals the connection between the SJ and GB meridians. The relationship between these meridians is further demonstrated when we understand that SJ 5 is the opening point for the Yang Wei, which has crossing points on the GB meridian at GB 13 – GB 21, and GB 35. Since Wei Guan is the luo-connecting point for the SJ, we have yet another demonstration of how luo points influence more than just their system three connections.

Internal Wind

This circuit is also useful when internal wind is present, and as traditional theory teaches us this pattern is rooted in a liver imbalance. Internal wind may be classified as either liver yang rising, liver wind, or liver blood/yin deficiency. This circuit should be used whenever internal wind presents as a liver yang rising or liver wind pattern. However, in the cases of internal wind arising from either a blood or yin deficiency, there may be more primary causative factors than just a liver imbalance. For instance, when liver blood deficiency has been diagnosed, it is helpful to look deeper into the pattern to see if the spleen and heart are involved in the pathogenesis. This can happen since the spleen and heart are the primary organs of blood production. This being the case, when blood deficiency is found to underlie internal wind, one should clearly differentiate between a prevalence of secondary symptoms affecting the liver, spleen, or heart. Since the SP and HT also connect to the shao yang, there will be some cases where it is preferable to use the shao yang-spleen/heart circuit over the shao yang-jue yin circuit. We shall examine this other circuit momentarily.

When a yin deficiency has been found as an underlying pattern effecting the shao yang, it is important to determine to what extent the kidneys are involved. Since the liver and kidneys share the same source, and both connect to the shao yang, it is important to determine which of these organs is most out of balance. If the secondary complaints indicate more of a kidney imbalance the shao yang-shao yin circuit should be emphasized.

SHAO YANG – SHAO YIN CIRCUIT

GB - SJ
-     -
HT - KI

Functions:

1) Harmonizes the Shao Yang and Shao Yin.

2) Calms the Shen.

3) Clears Heat.

4) Subdues Rising Yang, Fire, and Qi.

Primary Complaints: Neck pain, headaches, sciatica, hip pain, symptoms in the shao yang, fever, heat sensations.

2ⁿᵈ or 3ʳᵈ Concerns: Anxiety, insomnia, anemia, poor memory, palpitations, bone diseases, low back pain, infertility, low energy, hot flashes, and knee pain.

> " The manifestation of the shao yang channel is pain in the chest and rib area caused by pathogens, especially those originating in the gallbladder. This condition can affect the heart channel..."
> *Chapter 49, Nei Jing*

Explanation:

In the shao yang - shao yin circuit we observe the primary symptoms within the shao yang, and secondary complaints relating to the kidneys or heart.   This may include palpitations, stuffiness or pain in the chest, insomnia, poor memory, anemia, shen disturbance, low back pain, genital-urinary conditions, and reproductive diseases. This circuit is often used when shao yang symptoms present with underlying kidney yin deficiency, heart yin deficiency, or excessive heart fire.

When symptoms affect the shao yang it is important to assess the relative health of the kidneys. If the kidney yin is deficient, it can lead to symptoms associated with empty heat or liver yang rising, and these patterns will often affect the shao yang channels.

The Shao Yang and the Kidneys

The san jiao's association with the kidneys is widely recognized in traditional theory, as it is said that one of its functions to transport kidney yang to the rest of the body. Like the kidneys, the san jiao meridian also plays a major role in water metabolism, and it is the from the kidney yang that the san jiao derives its ability to transport water.

In regards to the gallbladder, the kidney is often involved when sciatic pain affects the GB channel. In addition, we find numerous associations between the KI and GB in the following points: GB 25 (Front Mu of the KI), GB 39 (Influential Point for Marrow), and GB 41 (Opening Point for the Dai).

The kidneys connection to the ear, as well as the location of SJ 21 and GB 2, is another important relationship between the shao yang and the kidneys.

When the shao yang has been determined to be the most important meridian pair to work with, it is essential to assess whether there is a greater imbalance in the jue yin or shao yin. If shao yin patterns or symptoms appear in

84

the patient's presentations, it will determine the use of completely different points than if the jue yin are involved. For instance, Tung's points 11.06, 11.14, 11.15, and 11.20 are all located on the ring finger and are therefore associated with the san jiao. While all of these points influence the liver, 11.14 and 11.20 have a greater effect on the liver, and 11.06 and 11.15 have a stronger influence on the kidneys. Therefore, choosing the best SJ and GB points to use is largely determined by the predominance of shao yin or jue yin root patterns.

Internal Wind

As discussed the shao yang is a major meridian pair to use for conditions of internal wind. In the previous circuit we reviewed how internal wind is attributed to either liver yang rising, liver wind, or a yin/blood deficiency. In cases of yin deficiency it should be determined if there is a predominance of liver or kidney signs. If the kidney signs and symptoms dominate, or if the client's secondary concern has to do with a kidney pattern, the shao yang -shao yin circuit should be emphasized over the shao yang-jue yin circuit. This is important to consider because we need to understand the etiology of the disease if we are to treat the root pattern. We shall continue this discussion after we have reviewed the next circuit that deals more with internal wind due to blood deficiency.

SHAO YANG – EARTH AND FIRE CIRCUIT

GB - SJ
- -
HT - SP

Functions:

1) Regulates the Shao Yang.

2) Benefits Blood Production and Circulation.

3) Treats Internal Wind from Blood Deficiency.

4) Influences Digestive Functions.

Primary Complaints: Headaches, neck and shoulder tension, symptoms in the shao yang channels, epilepsy, Parkinson's disease.

2nd and 3rd Concerns: Chest pain or stuffiness, anemia, dizziness, low appetite, bloating, edema, palpitations, heart disease.

Explanation:

For conditions where this circuit is to be used look for primary symptoms that involve the shao yang channels, and secondary complaints affecting the digestion, blood, heart, and circulation. This circuit is especially important when there are shao yang symptoms with spleen, heart, and blood deficiencies. When the blood is deficient it can cause wind and yang qi to rise and this will adversely affect the shao yang meridians. For this reason, we can treat the branch symptoms through the SJ and GB, while we treat the root pattern through nourishing the blood by strengthening the spleen and heart.

There are also numerous conditions that present with primary symptoms affecting the shao yang, but the condition is rooted in excessive heart fire. Temple headaches that occur with symptoms such as insomnia, hypertension, tongue sores, anger, palpitations, and heat sensations are one example. When heart fire underlies the presentation of shao yang symptoms SP 3, SP 4, and KI 2 is a good point combination that is often enough to treat the root pattern. These points overlap with Tung's points 66.10, 66.11, and 66.12, which are indicated for dizziness, blurred vision, hypertension, headaches, and palpitations due to heart fire. These points may also be used for imbalance between the kidney water and heart fire.

The Spleen and Heart

The connection between the spleen and heart occurs through their mutual influences on the blood, as well as their positions in the 5-element cycle. The strong association between these organs is clearly demonstrated in the functions of numerous spleen points. We have already mentioned SP 3 and SP 4 for their ability to clear heart fire, and SP 6 and SP 10 are both known for their ability to supplement and move blood. Although these functions are widely known, it is helpful to remember this in regards to the spleen's system five connection to the heart. Doing this can help one to see deeper into complex patterns.

The Etiology of Internal Wind Due to Blood Deficiency

Although it is common to think of internal wind as arising from a liver blood deficiency, we must not overlook the role the heart and spleen play in the development of a blood deficiency pattern. The liver does not stand alone in its presentations and imbalances, and since the spleen and heart are the primary organs of blood production, their role in the etiology and pathogenesis of blood deficient wind conditions needs to be ascertained. Simply identifying internal wind as coming from a liver blood deficiency does little to address any root imbalances that may underlie the deficiency.

Three Patterns of Internal Wind in the Shao Yang Channels

When using the shao yang to treat symptoms associated with internal wind it is important to understand the root causes. Traditionally internal wind is explained as either liver yang rising, liver wind, or liver yin/blood deficiency. Keeping with this traditional explanation, we find that the use of the shao yang - jue yin circuit is able to account for the basic pattern of internal wind coming from liver imbalances. However, if we look deeper into the etiology of internal wind, we find that liver yang rising and liver yin deficiency may in fact be due to an underlying kidney deficiency. A similar situation exists in regards to liver blood deficiency, since the spleen and heart are the primary organs of blood production.

For these reasons it is crucial to make a distinction between using the jue yin, shao yin, and spleen/heart circuits when treating internal wind. The final decision on what circuit to use depends on the patient's secondary and tertiary concerns, and secondarily on traditional methods of pattern identification. For instance, if a patient presents with a primary concern of temple headaches with eye twitches, a secondary concern of bloating after eating, and she has a pale puffy tongue, it would be most appropriate to use the shao yang - spleen/heart circuit. However, if the patient presents with a secondary concern of low back pain, we would most likely want to use the shao yang - shao yin circuit. If the client presents with a primary complaint related to internal wind, and has a secondary concern of headaches behind the eyes that occur with stress, the use of the shao yang - jue yin circuit would be optimum.

The key point in deciding what circuit to use is dictated by the patient's health priorities as determined by their primary, secondary, and tertiary complaints. Using this method of prioritizing their concerns allows the doctor to put the patient's needs first, rather than identifying traditional patterns that may not accurately reflect the patient's priorities in regards to their symptomatic presentations.

Given the complex etiology of a pattern such as internal wind, we will find cases where the primary complaint occurs in the shao yang, but the root pattern is more difficult to determine. It may be the case that we cannot clearly identify the liver or kidney patterns of yin deficiency. Likewise, we may not be able to determine whether a blood deficiency is rooted more in the liver, spleen, or heart. In such cases, and depending on the patients priorities and presentations, we may want to use a six meridian (6M) circuit as presented on the next page.

For Internal Wind with LV and KI Yin Deficiency	For Internal Wind with LV, SP, and HT Blood Deficiency
KI - HT - - SJ - GB - - PC - LV	SP - HT - - SJ - GB - - PC - LV

The above diagrams demonstrate how we may form 6M circuits when we add a meridian pair to a 4M circuit. Although this can be a valuable thing to do in complex patterns such as internal wind, it is usually best to work with 4M circuits. By doing so we are more clearly differentiating the primary imbalances and root patterns.

A Final Note on Internal Wind and Pattern Identification

The explanations on treating internal wind demonstrate how the use of meridian systems theory can lead us to the same conclusion's we would arrive at using traditional methods of pattern identification. The advantage of including a meridian based approach to differentiation is that it allows us to prioritize the patient's needs by accounting for their top symptomatic concerns. Systems theory allows us to be guided by the patient's *unique* presentations, rather than identifying them with a standard textbook pattern that may not adequately apply to their needs. When these methods are applied in clinical situations it often makes the work of pattern identification much easier.

CHAPTER 6

THE YIN CIRCUITS

As we move into discussing the next set of circuits it will be noticed that some of them have already been discussed in a slightly different context. For instance, when we talk about the tai yang - tai yin circuit, it is essentially the same as the tai yin - tai yang circuit; after all the exact same meridians are involved. The reason we distinguish between these has to do with the patient's primary and secondary complaints. If a patient's primary concern is neck and shoulder tension in the tai yang channels, but secondarily suffers from low energy and sluggish digestion, it is appropriate to think of the circuit as a tai yang – tai yin circuit. Conversely, if the client's two major concerns are digestive and respiratory symptoms, with a tertiary concern of neck tension along the UB channel, it is most advantageous to think of the circuit as a tai yin - tai yang circuit. In other words, the primary concern governs which meridian pair we prioritize, and the secondary concerns help us to determine what circuit is most appropriate to the overall treatment strategies. This is important because it helps us to identify the primary symptomatic meridians, as well as gain greater insight into root causes. This can help us to unravel complex patterns and arrive at better treatment strategies, and ultimately this method can guide us in selecting the most appropriate points to use.

As an example of why it is important to think of the tai yin - tai yang, and tai yang - tai yin circuits as being different, let's look at the various connections that can be formed with each of these pairs.

Tai Yin (LU - SP) Connects to:	Tai Yang (UB - SI) Connects to:
UB - SI	LU - SP
LI - ST	KI - HT
LV - SI	LU - LV

Even though the tai yin and tai yang connect to each other, the tai yin links with two other meridian pairs that the tai yang is not associated with. By prioritizing meridian pairs that are responsible for the client's chief concern, and then adding secondary pairs based on their other needs, we are identifying the main meridians and organs that are out of balance. This will allow us to more clearly differentiate patterns that are present, determine roots and branches, and refine our treatment strategy and point selections. For these reasons some of the circuits we will discuss in the following section are similar to ones we have previously covered.

TAI YIN: LU – SP

Functions:

1) Governs and Regulates Qi through Respiration and Digestion.

2) Tonifies Post-Natal Qi.

3) Regulates Fluid and Water Metabolism.

4) Benefits Wei Qi.

Whenever concurrent digestive and respiratory symptoms dominate a patient's clinical presentations it is appropriate to think of the tai yin system. In addition, the tai yin dominates many patterns of fatigue, water retention, low energy, depression, and poor immunity.

The tai yin meridians may be paired with three other meridian pairs: the tai yang, yang ming, and the liver and small intestine. These circuits are represented as:

SP - LU	SP - LU	SP - LU
- -	- -	- -
SI - UB	ST - LI	SI - LV

When the tai yin has been identified as the primary meridians to be treated, one must then determine whether they should be paired with the tai yang, yang ming, or the liver and small intestine. Choosing which meridians to pair the tai yin with is determined by the patient's secondary concerns, or the underlying pattern that is present. If a patient's primary complaint is low energy with asthma, and the secondary concern is chronic loose stools, it would be appropriate to choose the tai yin - yang ming circuit. With a primary concern of low immunity, a secondary concern of bloating, and a tertiary concern of neck and back pain, choose the tai yin - tai yang circuit. Similarly, if the patient presents with shortness of breath and chest tightness, a secondary concern of hepatitis, and has a third concern of low appetite, it would be best to work with the tai yin - liver/small intestine circuit. Let's now examine each of these circuits in detail.

TAI YIN – TAI YANG CIRCUIT

LU - SP
-      -
UB - SI

Functions:

1) Governs Qi through Respiration and Digestion.

2) Regulates Water and Fluid Metabolism.

3) Benefits Wei Qi.

Primary Complaints: Asthma, bronchitis, sinusitis, allergies, weak appetite, poor digestion, bloating, diarrhea, low energy, immune deficiency.

2nd or 3rd Concerns: Neck, back, shoulder, and spinal pain, neurological conditions, headaches, bladder diseases.

Explanation:

The tai yin - tai yang circuit is to be used when the patient's chief complaints involve the tai yin and secondary symptoms relate to the tai yang. This will present as respiratory or digestive conditions with secondary or tertiary concerns in the tai yang channels. Typical zang-fu patterns for this circuit include qi deficiency, spleen damp, cold invasions of the lungs, and lung phlegm accumulation.

When damp accumulation effects the spleen and lungs, it can be useful to work with the tai yang due to their role in separating and excreting fluids. If dampness has invaded the lungs the joint combination of LU 5 and UB 40 are a powerful combination. Lung 5 is the water point on the lung meridian and has the function of descending fluids to the UB. Urinary bladder 40 is the earth point on a water meridian, it helps to regulate water metabolism, and also has a strong effect on the metal energy of the lungs and skin.

Immunity, Wei Qi, and the Lungs and Spleen

When immune deficiency has roots in the tai yin it is essential to supplement the lungs and spleen. In addition, since the tai yang is associated with the superficial regions of the body, and has a direct connection to the wei qi, it is always important to determine the relative health of the tai yang in immune deficient conditions. Since the tai yang directly connects to the tai yin, they are instrumental in many patterns of immune deficiency, especially when secondary symptoms effect the UB or SI meridians. The use of the urinary bladder back-shu points are essential in treating these types of patterns.

The Tai Yin in the Treatment of Neck and Back Pain

On the LU meridian we find a number of points that are indicated for symptoms affecting the neck and back along the UB channel. The most well known point is LU 7, which is commonly indicated for neck stiffness due to wind cold invasion. However, since the LU and UB connect in system two, LU 7 may be used for any pattern of neck pain that occurs along the UB meridian.

In Tung's acupuncture methods we find numerous points on the LU meridian that treat neck, back, and lumbar pain. Xiao Jie (A.05) is located at the distal portion of the first metacarpal bone about 1 cun distal to LU 10, it is indicated for pain in the neck, shoulders, back, and lumbar regions. Similarly, the points Chong Zi (22.10) and Chong Shen (22.02) are located on the thenar eminence and are very useful for neck and upper back pain.

Ren Shi (33.13) is located on the lung meridian 4 cun above the wrist crease and is indicated for pain in the upper back. Related to this, I have found it very useful to needle any reactive points, 1 - 5 cun proximal to LU 7, when there is pain in the scapular and thoracic regions.

On the spleen meridian, SP 3 has been indicated by some sources for strengthening the spine, while 77.17 (SP 9) is used in Tung acupuncture to treat tightness in the neck and thoracic area. Similarly, Shen Guan (77.18) is located 1.5 cun below SP 9, and it is known to treat shoulder conditions. The ability of this point for treating the shoulders can be understood because the SP connects to both the LU and SI, both of which pass through the shoulder.

TAI YIN – YANG MING CIRCUIT

SP - LU

-       -

ST - LI

Functions:

1) Governs Qi through Respiration and Digestion.

2) Benefits the Stomach and Intestines.

3) Regulates Bowel Functions.

Primary Concerns: Weak digestion, bloating, chronic diarrhea, fatigue, PMS, asthma, cough, shortness of breath, bronchitis.

2nd or 3rd Concerns: Diarrhea, constipation, sinusitis, PMS, abdominal pain, deficient stomach acid.

Explanation:

The use of this circuit will depend on primary symptoms that involve the tai yin, and secondary or tertiary concerns that are connected to the yang ming. This is an earth-metal circuit that has broad applications in a variety of respiratory and digestive conditions. This includes food allergies, Candida, asthma, immune deficiency, and external invasions that affect the lungs and digestive systems.

Qi deficiency of the lungs and spleen is often treated with this circuit, and it is usually the first choice when there are numerous digestive symptoms present. When qi deficiency of the lungs and spleen exist the simultaneous use of LI 10 and ST 36 is a powerful combination, and these two points are an example of mirroring in the yang ming meridians.

If the primary condition effects the spleen rather than the lungs, this circuit is appropriate to use if there are also lung symptoms present. If a patient's primary concern is low energy with poor appetite and digestion, and the secondary concern involves the respiratory system, this circuit should be used.

This is not the only circuit to use for spleen pattern digestive conditions, if the patient presents with a primary concern of low energy and poor appetite, and has a secondary concern of palpitations, it would be best to use another circuit. Similarly, if a patient's chief concern was low energy with a poor appetite, and their secondary concern was pain in the neck and shoulders along the tai yang meridians, it would be most appropriate to use the tai yin - tai yang circuit. This method of prioritizing a patient's top three health concerns, helps us to identify what meridian systems and circuits should be used in developing the treatment protocol.

Stomach Points that Influence the Lungs

In TCM styles of acupuncture we find two stomach points that are often used to treat lung conditions. Stomach 36 is used in cases of lung qi deficiency and asthma, and ST 40 is used for phlegm in the lungs. In Tung style acupuncture the points 77.08, 77.09, 77.10 are located on the ST meridian and are indicated for asthma and numerous other lung conditions. Similarly, the points 88.17, 88.18, and 88.19, are also used for a variety of lung syndromes and dermatological conditions.

Lung Points for the Digestion

Tu Shui (22.11) located on the lung meridian at the thenar muscle, is indicated for a variety of patterns involving the stomach and spleen. The name itself translates as Earth-Water, and is therefore called for when there is damp accumulation causing loose stool or diarrhea. It is also indicated for gastropathy and stomachaches.

Food Allergies and Candida

This is usually the primary circuit to work with for conditions of food allergies and Candida. This is because these diseases often involve both the digestive and respiratory systems. Some of the most common symptoms of food allergies are abdominal bloating or pain, nausea, diarrhea, nasal congestion, difficulty breathing, and skin conditions such as hives, itching, and eczema. Many of these same symptoms are also present with Candida, and it is evident that these symptoms clearly point to a primary imbalance in the tai yin - yang ming circuit. In zang-fu pattern identification we often classify these conditions as spleen and lung deficiency with damp or phlegm accumulation.

TAI YIN – WOOD AND FIRE CIRUIT

LU - SP

-   -

LV - SI

Functions:

1) Governs Qi through Respiration and Digestion.

2) Controls the Dispersion, Circulation, and Smooth Flow of Qi.

3) Benefits Wei Qi.

4) Influences Water, Fluid, and Blood Metabolism.

Primary Complaints: Respiratory and digestive diseases, coughing, chest tightness, loss of appetite, bloating, edema, abdominal pain, diarrhea, and fatigue.

2nd and 3rd Concerns: Headaches, hepatitis, jaundice, PMS, shoulder or scapular tension, stress, irritability.

Explanation:

This circuit is useful when liver patterns are effecting the respiration or digestion, and is also causing pain in the upper back, shoulders, and SI channel. When liver qi stagnation overacts on the lungs it leads to tightness in the chest, cough, and other respiratory symptoms. When it overacts on the spleen it can cause abdominal pain, loss of appetite, bloating, and other spleen related symptoms. Liver qi stagnation also commonly effects the neck and shoulders, and since the LV and SI are linked in system four, we can easily understand how liver stagnation can cause pain in the scapular, shoulders, and neck.

The Role of Metal, in Liver Overacting on Spleen Patterns

In patterns where the liver is overacting on the spleen and causing abdominal pain or other symptoms, it can be very helpful to use lung points. This is especially true if lung symptoms are also present. Needling the LU meridian also allows us to use metal to counterbalance excessive wood energy. For abdominal complaints due to liver overacting on the spleen, use LU 5 and LU 7 in combination on one side. In addition to the metal-wood dynamics, LU 7 opens the RN and can regulate the qi in the lower abdomen and three jiaos. In imaging, LU 5 is associated with the navel region, and is therefore beneficial for abdominal conditions. In systems theory, the lung meridian influences the RN, SP, and LV channels, all of which pass through the abdomen. This makes the use of LU 5 and LU 7 important for liver patterns that are simultaneously effecting the lungs, spleen, and abdomen.

Wood – Fire – Earth (LV – SI – SP)

The presence of the SI meridian in this circuit can be understood in terms of 5-elements. Since the SI is a fire meridian, it may be used to reduce the wood of the liver, while boosting the spleen and earth functions. There are numerous points on the SI channel that are used for treating liver conditions. For example, SI 4 is an empirical point for jaundice, and SI 7 the luo-connecting point, is known to treat emotional conditions of the wood element. Also located on the SI meridian are Tung's points Chang

102

Men (33.10) and Gan Men (33.11), which are both indicated for enteritis due to acute hepatitis. In addition, 33.10 is indicated for diarrhea and abdominal cramps. In the above examples the ability of the SI points may be understood in two ways. First, the SI connects to the liver in system four, and second, it connects to the spleen in system two. As just shown, the above points reduce excess liver conditions and assist the spleen in transforming dampness.

SI 5, Fire on Fire, Tai Yang and the Neck

Small intestine 5 is a fire point on a fire meridian, it is useful for reducing excess in the wood element, and strengthening the earth energies. In addition, since the wrist images the neck it is also useful for tai yang pattern neck pain. Use this point for liver-spleen patterns that also present with neck, shoulder, and scapular pain in the tai yang channels. This point combines well with SI 3 when the pain is located in the neck.

A useful point combination for shoulder and scapular pain in the SI channel, with an underlying liver imbalance, is SI 6, SI 7, LV 3, LV 4, and LV 5. Needling the SI meridian on the same side as the pain invigorates the circulation through the channel. In addition, SI 7 and LV 5 are both the luo-connecting points, and when these points are needled together, they allow the meridians to communicate with one another. For best results first needle the LV points to address the underlying condition and follow by needling the SI points. For pain along the SI meridian in the region of the shoulder blades or neck, SI 3, SI 5, and SI 6 are good choices. Choose SI 3 and SI 5 when the pain is closer to the neck, and SI 6 when it is in the scapula.

SHAO YIN: HT - KI

Functions:

1) Governs Blood and Essence.

2) Calms the Shen.

3) Maintains the Essential Balance between Fire and Water, Yin and Yang.

4) Controls Fluid Metabolism.

The shao yin organs and meridians of the heart and kidneys are associated with the blood and essence. These are the most vital fluids of the body and are connected with reproduction, the marrow, and the higher nervous system functions of the mind and spirit. Since the blood is the root of the mind, and the heart houses the shen, the functions of the heart are deeply connected to consciousness. Just as important as the blood and heart are to conscious activity, is the kidney essence and functions of the marrow and Ming Men. The marrow that fills the brain and spinal cord is an essential aspect of development and consciousness, and the Ming Men is connected to our spiritual purpose and destiny. The connection between the vital fluids of the blood and essence, and the spirit and destiny, are all contained within the fundamental relationship between the fire and water of the heart and kidneys. This is the essence and vitality of the shao yin.

The shao yin combines with three other meridian pairs including the tai yang, shao yang, and the spleen and san jiao. Each of these circuits are listed on the next page.

HT - KI	HT - KI	HT - KI
- -	- -	- -
SI - UB	GB - SJ	SP - SJ

When working with the shao yin secondary symptoms need to be accurately accounted for. When the secondary concerns indicate a tai yang imbalance it is best to use the shao yin - tai yang circuit. If shao yin imbalances occur with temple headaches, internal wind, or conditions along the GB and SJ meridians, it is often best to use the shao yin - shao yang circuit. When there is a shao yin disharmony with digestive symptoms, hormonal imbalance, or blood deficiency, it is preferable to use the shao yin - spleen/san jiao circuit. Let's now examine these circuits in greater detail.

SHAO YIN – TAI YANG CIRCUIT

HT - KI
- -
SI - UB

FUNCTIONS:

1) Governs Blood and Essence.

2) Influences the Head, Neck, Shoulders, and Spine.

3) Controls Water and Fluid Metabolism.

4) Regulates Fluid Separation and Excretion.

Primary Concerns: Heart and kidney diseases, shen disturbance, insomnia, anxiety, depression, palpitations, poor memory, infertility, impotence, frigidity, anemia.

2nd and 3rd Concerns: Neck, back, shoulder, and spinal pain, urinary bladder diseases, edema.

Explanation:

When imbalances exist in the heart or kidneys it can easily effect the externally related meridians of the small intestine and urinary bladder. This circuit is to be used when the primary concern involves the heart or kidneys, and the tai yang are also involved. Look for conditions such as palpitations, shen disturbance, fatigue, infertility, and kidney diseases; that occur with neck, back, shoulder, or lumbar pain.

106

Elementally, this circuit deals with fire and water balance. Disharmony between these elements are often associated with various patterns of shen disturbance, and when these types of conditions occur it is often necessary to restore the balance between the heart and kidneys. Since the heart circulates the blood and houses the spirit, it has a strong influence on one's overall state of consciousness. When the heart's functions are taken into consideration with the kidneys role in producing and storing marrow, we can understand how this circuit is important for mental, emotional, and neurological conditions. While both the shen of the heart, and the Ming Men of the kidneys, strongly influence the conscious aspects of being, the tai yang is closely associated with the physical aspects of the spine, brain, and nervous system. Taken together these four meridians are fundamental for treating conditions involving the mind, emotions, and neurological system.

Heart Patterns

This circuit can be useful for a number of heart patterns including heart yin deficiency, heart qi or yang deficiency, and water accumulation effecting the heart. For these patterns, the kidneys are usually involved and they play an important role in the etiology of the disease. With the fundamental connection between the shao yin organs, it is often necessary to consider the relative health of the kidneys in many heart patterns.

For patterns such as heart qi and yang deficiency, or when water accumulation influences the heart, the tai yang also play an important role in the supplementation of heart energies.

In cases of water accumulation effecting the heart, it may be the case that the shao yin - spleen/san jiao circuit is involved. To determine what circuit to use the patient's top concerns and presenting symptoms should be determined. In cases of spleen signs and symptoms it is best to use the shao yin - SP/SJ circuit; however, if spinal conditions or bladder symptoms present, use the shao yin - tai yang circuit.

Blood and Essence

In cases of blood and essence deficiency this circuit should be considered; however, this will depend on the patient's manifestations and priorities. If kidney essence deficiency presents with back and spinal conditions effecting the tai yang, this circuit would be an appropriate choice. However, it is possible that an essence deficiency could produce symptoms in the shao yang, rather than the tai yang. In this case it would be best to use the shao yin - shao yang circuit. Let's now examine the properties of this circuit in more detail.

SHAO YIN – SHAO YANG CIRCUIT

HT - KI
-    -
GB - SJ

Functions:

1) Governs Blood and Essence.

2) Transports Qi, Blood, and Essence to the Head.

3) Benefits the Ear.

4) Clears Heat.

Primary Concerns: Low back pain, osteoporosis, sciatica, infertility, palpitations, anxiety, fear, restlessness, shen disturbance, insomnia, dizziness, Parkinson's disease.

2nd and 3rd Concerns: Temple headaches, sciatica in the GB channel, neck and shoulder tension, fever.

Explanation:

The shao yin - shao yang circuit is used when primary signs and symptoms exist in the shao yin, and secondary concerns involve the shao yang. When the heart or kidneys become deficient, it can often influence the shao yang and lead to symptoms such as temple headaches and GB meridian sciatica. When the heart blood/yin is deficient, it can cause the vessels to constrict, and lead to headaches in the GB channel. Heart blood/yin deficiencies are also associated with insomnia, and when sleeplessness occurs with temple headaches, it is often a good choice to use a circuit that contains both the GB and HT.

Though the KI and GB are not directly connected, sciatica in the GB channel is often associated with a kidney deficiency. In these cases the root treatment should focus on nourishing the kidneys, while the branch aspect of the treatment can see good results by needling SJ points on the opposite side of the pain. Points on the SJ meridian such as SJ 3, SJ 5, and SJ 6, are indicated for back pain, and are most effective when the GB meridian is involved. In Tung style acupuncture there are many points on the SJ meridian that are indicated for low back pain and sciatica of the GB channel, these include: 11.15, 22.06, 22.07, 33.07, and 44.02.

Heart Fire and the Shao Yang

Excessive heart fire is associated with mouth and tongue sores, as well as symptoms that involve the shao yang. These include symptoms such as anger, constipation, heat sensations, and insomnia. When heart fire is present it is often necessary to use this circuit, as the SJ helps to clear heat and relive constipation. The GB channel is helpful for relieving anger, clearing heat, and assisting in treating insomnia. In cases of heart fire causing temple headaches, it is also important to use GB points on the foot. The use of this circuit in treating heart fire is dependent on secondary or tertiary complaints that involve the shao yang.

Shao Yin Roots, Shao Yang Branches

In many conditions involving this circuit the shao yin will be responsible for the root disharmony, and the shao yang will manifest the branch symptoms. When the primary concern involves the heart or kidneys, take careful consideration for what the patient's second and third concerns are. This is vital to determining the most appropriate circuits and points to use.

In any style of acupuncture there are numerous points that may be selected for any given condition. The key to getting the most effective point combinations is often determined by identifying not only the pattern that is present, but also the patient's top symptomatic concerns. This is in contrast to traditional methods of pattern differentiation that take the primary symptom as the starting point, and then look for other signs and symptoms to confirm a zang-fu pattern. This way of proceeding can easily allow for too much subjectivity on part of the therapist. For example, it is all too common that a client will complain of a temple headache, and the doctor will immediately look for a confirmation that a liver pattern exists. This usually isn't hard to find, but this approach does not necessarily identify the core pattern of disharmony, or the patient's other health priorities. The patient with temple headaches and a secondary concern of heart disease, can easily get misdiagnosed as a liver pattern, when in actuality the primary disharmony involves the shao yin - shao yang circuit. By asking the patient to prioritize their needs we are better able to identify the most problematic conditions the patient has. If we don't ask the patient what their secondary and tertiary concerns are, we may never know, and one could easily end up focusing on a related, but less important pattern. This will deduce the effectiveness of our treatment strategies and point combinations.

SHAO YIN – SPLEEN AND SAN JIAO CIRCUIT

HT - KI

\- \-

SP - SJ

Functions:

1) Governs Blood and Essence.

2) Governs Yin and Yang, Fire and Water.

3) Distributes Kidney Yang through the San Jiao.

4) Regulates Blood and Fluid Metabolism.

Primary Symptoms: Low back pain, edema, impotence, water swelling, anemia, palpitations, dizziness, tinnitus, infertility, heart and kidney diseases, shen disturbance.

2nd and 3rd Concerns: Diarrhea, low appetite, bloating, digestive weakness, water retention, fatigue.

Explanation:

In this circuit it is very useful to think in terms of 5-elements since fire, earth, and water are all present. The fire is represented by both the heart and san jiao, the earth by the spleen, and the water by the kidneys. Excesses or deficiencies in either of these elements can easily effect one another and lead to a number of complex patterns. As an example, a deficiency in the spleen can lead to blood deficiency in the heart, and if prolonged can even cause an essence deficiency in the kidneys.

In longstanding cases of blood or essence deficiency it can be difficult to ascertain the etiology. If an imbalance started in the spleen, and then led to a blood deficiency, this can drain the kidney essence since 'the blood and essence share the same source.' This condition will then effect the other organs and create further imbalance. Alternately, a deficiency in the kidney may effect the spleen, and over time lead to a spleen and heart blood deficiency. When either of these patterns has been present for a prolonged amount of time it will lead to complicated cases and multiple zang-fu patterns.

By using the shao yin - spleen/san jiao circuit we are able to address these types of branch and root conditions, simultaneously, without having the difficult task of determining the etiological processes and multiple zang-fu patterns that may be present. By taking a meridian based approach it becomes much easier to ascertain complex patterns and get quick and efficient results. The proof of this comes through the experience of working this system on thousands of clients.

Heart and Spleen

The connection between the spleen and heart it well known, not only in 5-elements, but also in the role that these two organs share in blood production. If the spleen is deficient, and the blood production is compromised, it can easily effect the heart. Heart and spleen blood deficiency is a common pattern, as is the use of spleen points for conditions of heart blood deficiency or stagnation. Spleen points that are commonly selected for various heart patterns include: SP 6, SP 10, 66.10 (SP 3), 66.11 (SP 4), 77.17, and 77.18.

The San Jiao

The san jiao plays an important function in this circuit as it belongs to the fire element, and it transports yuan qi from the kidneys to the spleen. This is interesting because in meridian systems theory the SJ connects the spleen and kidneys. Although using the SJ as a fire organ to strengthen the spleen is not widely practiced, it makes sense when we consider its role in transporting kidney yang to the spleen. Since the SJ also regulates the water passages, we find that it serves a triple function in benefiting the spleen. First, it belongs to the fire element, secondly it transports kidney yang to the spleen, and finally it functions to regulate the water passages. All of these functions make the SJ important for regulating activities of the spleen, when the kidneys are also involved in the overall pattern. The ability of the SJ meridian to regulate the spleen's functions, through the kidneys, is indicated in the points SJ 4 and 11.21. It is also worth mentioning that in some forms of Japanese acupuncture SJ 5 is commonly used with moxa in cases of spleen and kidney yang deficiency.

Spleen 4, The Chong Mai and the Kidneys

Though the spleen and kidneys are not directly connected in meridian systems theory, they are linked through the heart and san jiao in this circuit. In traditional theory we also find a strong association between the spleen and kidney through the Chong mai, as it should be remembered that this extra-ordinary meridian has crossing points with KI 11 - KI 21. This makes SP 4 a powerful point for opening kidney points in the abdomen. In addition, one of the functions of the Chong mai is to connect the pre and post-natal qi, and this is yet another demonstration of the relationship between the SP and KI.

In Tung style acupuncture we find many points that are located on the SP meridian that strongly benefit the kidney functions. For instance, 77.17, 77.18, 77.19, 88.09, 88.10, and 88.11 are all indicated for deficiency conditions of the spleen and kidneys.

Damp Accumulation Due to Spleen and Kidney Deficiency

This circuit can be useful for various conditions involving damp accumulation due to deficiencies in the spleen and kidneys. While the KI and SP meridians play a primary role in the treatment of this pattern, the san jiao plays an important adjunct role since it functions to transport water and kidney yang. Since it is a fire meridian it may be used for either damp cold or damp heat patterns.

Points located on the SJ meridian that are recognized in Tung style acupuncture such as 11.15, 33.04, 33.05, and 33.06 are also useful in treating certain heart and chest disorders. While 11.15 and 33.04 are used for palpitations, 33.05 and 33.06 are indicated for pain and distension in the chest. This may be understood in terms of the connection between the SJ and PC, but these points may be used for heart conditions when this circuit is indicated due to underlying imbalances in the spleen and kidneys.

Spleen Points for the Heart and Kidneys

We have already covered numerous spleen points that are good for the heart, for review these are 66.10 (SP 3), 66.11 (SP 4), SP 6, and SP 10. In Tung style acupuncture SP 3, SP 4, and KI 2 are used in combination to clear heart heat, and they restore balance between the heart and kidneys; they may also be used in the treatment of palpitations and hypertension. Similarly, Master Tung used 77.17 (SP 9) for heart diseases, hypertension, and other heart related conditions, and this point is also commonly used for water accumulation due to spleen and kidney deficiencies.

Also on the spleen line are three of Master Tung's points that are used in the treatment of various diseases related to spleen and kidney deficiencies. These points are 77.18, 77.19, and 77.21 (SP 6), they all have the dual function of supplementing the spleen and kidneys. Since the SP and KI connect to the HT, these points are also very useful for patterns of damp accumulation that effect the heart, which are rooted in deficiencies of the spleen and kidneys.

In summary, this circuit is good for conditions involving the blood, abdomen, heart, spleen and kidneys. It is especially useful when there is concurrent deficiency in the spleen qi/ yang, heart blood, and kidney essence, or when there is damp accumulation involving these organs.

JUE YIN: LV - PC

Functions:

1) Regulates Circulation of Qi and Blood.

2) Calms the Shen.

3) Supplements Yin and Blood.

The jue yin is a major circuit for regulating circulation, nourishing yin and blood, and calming the mind and emotions. One of the primary functions of the liver is to maintain the free flow of qi, while the pericardium functions with the heart to circulate the blood. Taken together we may say that the jue yin is the major pair for circulating both the qi and blood. In coordination with the pericardium's function of circulating blood, is the liver's role in storing blood. Given the strong connection that each of these organs has with the blood, and the pericardium's connection to the Yin Wei and Chong meridians, we should carefully consider these organs in any condition that involves blood. In contrast to the heart and spleen that function in blood circulation and production, the liver and pericardium function in blood storage and circulation.

Another major function of the jue yin is to regulate and calm the shen. This is seen in the function of many pericardium points, and in the many ways in which liver imbalance can cause shen disturbance. When the jue yin are used together, and according to a patient's clinical presentations, it can be a powerful combination for releasing emotion held in the body. The jue yin are also especially effective for various mental and emotional imbalances that are caused by stress, and it is helpful to think of the jue yin as a stress buffer for the rest of the body. This corresponds to the pericardium's role of protecting the heart from pathological influences.

The circuits formed from the jue yin are:

LV - PC	LV - PC	LV - PC
- -	- -	- -
GB - SJ	LI - ST	LI - KI

Let's now review each of these circuits in detail.

JUE YIN – SHAO YANG CIRCUIT

LV - PC
- -
GB - SJ

Functions:

1) Regulates Circulation of Qi and Blood.

2) Subdues Liver Yang and Internal Wind.

3) Calms the Shen.

4) Clears Heat and Damp Heat.

Primary Concerns: Headaches, anxiety, tightness in the chest, insomnia, restlessness, stroke, hypertension, PMS, hepatitis.

2nd or 3rd Concerns: Hip pain, shen disturbance, temple headaches, heat sensations, any symptoms within the shao yang channels.

Explanation:

Liver disharmonies are some of the most common patterns observed in clinic, and provide a great opportunity for discussing the benefits of using meridian systems.   For each of the symptomatic expressions of liver imbalance, the points selected should correspond with the patient's *unique* presentations.   For instance, liver qi stagnation that manifests with headaches and neck pain should be treated differently than liver stagnation that is causing abdominal and digestive symptoms. When the patient suffers from temple headaches with pain behind the eyes it is usually most appropriate to use the jue yin - shao yang circuit. However, if the patient experiences abdominal pain with constipation and acid reflux, it would be best to use the jue yin - yang ming circuit.

Liver Imbalance and Headaches

There are several patterns of headaches that are related to liver imbalance, and these include headaches behind the eyes, at the vertex, temples, as well in the yang ming channels. Traditional theory teaches that since the liver connects to the eyes, and the liver channel extends to the vertex, pain at either of these locations is related to the liver. Temple headaches are usually associated with liver yang rising or liver fire, and yang ming headaches are often classified as damp, phlegm, or stomach patterns.

Taking a meridian based approach, temple headaches in the GB channel can be treated with SJ, HT, and LV points; while yang ming headaches that are rooted in an underlying liver imbalance are best treated with the LI meridian. This is because the LI connects to both the LV and ST channels.

For most conditions of the head and neck that are rooted in a liver pattern it is best to use the jue yin - shao yang circuit. This is because both the GB and SJ meridians transverse the head, and have numerous points that are useful for treating symptoms in the head and neck. The exception to this is when liver patterns cause symptoms in either the LI or ST channels. For these conditions it is best to use the jue yin - yang ming circuit which we will discuss in the next section.

Temple Headaches

The ability of circuit theory to integrate and account for various patterns of liver related temple headaches, is easily demonstrated by observing the numerous functions of the jue yin - shao yang circuit. Temple headaches and migraines may be identified as liver qi stagnation, liver fire, or liver yang rising, and regardless of the zang-fu differentiation, the jue yin - shao yang circuit may be applied. In the case of liver stagnation, the LV, PC, and GB meridians are all known to have the ability to resolve stagnant liver qi; while in cases of liver fire and liver yang rising, the SJ meridian is known to clear heat and subdue liver yang. For these various zang-fu patterns, the jue yin - shao yang circuit has the capacity to treat temple headaches that are rooted in various types of liver imbalances, and this demonstrates an important point we have been making throughout the book, which is:

Meridian Systems and 4M Circuits are often able to account for various zang-fu syndromes, as well as identify the most pertinent patterns of disharmony.

We just discussed how temple headaches may be due to various liver patterns, and how the jue yin - shao yang circuit is able to treat any of these zang fu syndromes. While temple headaches are often due to liver patterns, we should also remember that the shao yang connects to the shao yin, as well as to the heart and spleen. Therefore, there are cases that have a primary concern of temple headaches but do not manifest other liver signs. Since the shao yang also connects to the shao yin, it is possible that a patient could manifest more heart and kidney symptoms. If the blood, essence, or yin are deficient it can cause the vessels to constrict and result in pain in the temples. In this case the patient would manifest more signs and symptoms that indicate a greater imbalance in the shao yin.   Similarly, I have seen cases where the patient manifested temple headaches without any other liver signs or symptoms, and the secondary complaints and root pattern were related to a spleen and heart blood deficiency. Rather then using the jue yin - shao yang circuit in these cases, it is best to use the shao yang - SP/HT circuit.

For a majority of temple headaches the jue yin - shao yang circuit will be used, but this depends on there being a pre-dominance of liver signs and symptoms. The jue yin – shao yang circuit is also effectively used for a number of other head and neck conditions that are rooted in liver imbalances. This is because of the location of the GB and SJ meridians through the neck and head, as well as the ability of both GB and SJ points to resolve various liver patterns.

For conditions of the head SJ 1, SJ 2, SJ 3, and 11.14 are all good choices, on the GB meridian GB 41 - GB 44 are appropriate. These points can be understood by imaging the head to the hands and feet. For neck conditions with an underlying liver imbalance we find that SJ 3, SJ 4, SJ 5, GB 39, GB 40, and GB 42 are commonly indicated; this reveals the correspondence between imaging the distal end of the long bones to the neck.

JUE YIN - YANG MING CIRCUIT

LV - PC
-   -
LI - ST

Functions:

1) Regulates Circulation of Qi and Blood through the Digestive System.

2) Harmonizes the Stomach, Intestines, and Bowels.

3) Clears Heat.

Primary Concerns: Stress, headaches, IBS, palpitations, tightness in the chest, irritability, costal pain, hepatitis, liver diseases.

2nd or 3rd Concerns: Acid reflux, IBS, stomach and abdominal pains due to liver patterns, constipation, colitis, diarrhea, vomiting, nausea, ulcers.

Explanation:

This circuit is extremely useful for stomach and abdominal symptoms when liver disharmonies are the causative factor. This includes conditions such as IBS, acid reflux, constipation, abdominal pain, plum pit, abdominal masses, gynecological conditions, colitis, and ulcers.

In the last section we examined how the jue yin - shao yang circuit is useful for liver patterns that result in symptoms in the head and neck. In this circuit the jue yin connects with the yang ming, which has a strong influence on the abdomen. The contrast between these two circuits clearly demonstrates the importance of identifying not only traditional zang-fu patterns, but also the necessity of taking a meridian based approach. To elaborate, let's compare two cases that could easily be differentiated as a liver qi stagnation pattern.

In the first case the client suffers from headaches that are worse with stress and are primarily located behind the eyes. She also has tightness in the chest that is related to stress, and it occurs when she thinks about past painful situations. As a tertiary complaint she suffers from hip pain. The pulse is wiry.

In the second case the patient also suffers from headaches behind the eyes, but has a secondary concern of palpitations. Both of these symptoms are made worse with stress, and the patient also experiences frequent anxiety. The third complaint is abdominal pain, and the pulse is wiry.

For each of the cases liver qi stagnation can easily be identified from the patients top three concerns and pulse presentations. Potentially the same treatment could be given to each patient based on the syndrome differentiation of liver qi stagnation with a primary concern of headaches. However, if we are careful about our intake, questioning, and analysis of diseased meridians, we would find some differences. In the first case the headaches most often occur behind the eyes, but the temples are occasionally effected as well. With palpation we find that the hip pain is located in the region of GB 29 - GB 30.

In the second case the patient suffers from headaches behind the eyes and she occasionally feels them in the forehead. With palpation we find that the third complaint of abdominal pain is located on the ST meridian.

When we compare these cases we find that the first case experiences liver qi stagnation headaches with pain in the GB channel, and the hip pain also confirms the presence of an imbalance in the GB meridian. For this reason we decide to use the jue yin - shao yang circuit. In the second case, the headaches are also the priority, but the forehead and yang ming channels are involved. The patient's third concern of abdominal pain on the ST meridian also indicates that the yang ming are involved, and for this reason we decide to use the jue yin - yang ming circuit.

The above examples demonstrate why it is important to question the patient about their top three concerns, as well as identifying what meridians are expressing symptoms. While asking the patient to prioritize their concerns allows the therapist to sort through all the numerous symptoms the patient may have, it also allows for more accurate pattern identification. Identifying a zang-fu pattern and basing a treatment entirely on that does not necessarily account for the most pressing concerns the patient has, nor will it always lead to the best point prescriptions. In contrast, asking the patient about their priorities, and using meridian systems and circuit theory, greatly assists the therapist in refining the treatment strategy.

This method of reasoning is crucial if we are to maximize our results while using fewer needles. While zang-fu differentiation is a crucial aspect of pattern identification, it may not always allow for the finer discrimination of selecting only the most appropriate meridians and points. By taking a meridian based approach to syndrome differentiation, we are able to effectively determine zang-fu patterns, and select only the most relevant points that allow for the greatest effects.

The Pericardium, Liver Imbalance, and the Yang Ming

For many conditions where liver disharmony is causing yang ming symptoms the use of the PC meridian is very important. We have already covered this, and in summary the PC meridian is very effective for moving liver qi, harmonizing the stomach, and calming the mind. The last function of calming the mind is essential for many of the digestive and abdominal patterns where the cause is stress related or psychosomatic in origin.

It should be remembered that the PC connects with most of the major meridians flowing through the abdomen. It is linked with the KI, ST, and LV, as well as with the SP through the pairing of PC 6 and SP 4, the Yin Wei also has crossing points with SP 13, SP 15, and SP 16.

PC 6 and Plum Pit Syndrome

Keeping with the theory that the distal portions of the long bones image the neck and throat we find that PC 6 opens the Yin Wei, which terminates at Ren 22 and Ren 23. This makes the use of PC 6 an important point for plum pit qi. If we examine the traditional explanation for this syndrome it is explained as liver qi stagnation with phlegm. Reviewing the jue yin - yang ming circuit we find that it makes a perfect fit for addressing this problem. The liver and large intestine meridians treat the stagnation, ST points resolve phlegm, and PC 6 opens the Yin Wei, which connects with RN 22 and RN 23. In addition, the ST and LI meridians pass through the throat. A final point prescription looks as follows: LV 7, LV 3, Ling Ku on the left side; and PC 6, PC 7, ST 40, and ST 41 on the right side.

126

Gynecological Conditions

The jue yin - yang ming circuit is one of the major circuits used for gynecological conditions. Though there are various patterns involving other organ systems, the function of the liver in moving qi and storing blood plays a major role in many of these conditions. Large intestine points are also frequently used, and this can be understood due to the system two correspondences between the LI and LV. We will cover the ways in which this circuit may be used for treating dysmenorrhea in a later section.

THE JUE YIN – METAL AND WATER CIRCUIT

$$LV - PC$$
$$- \quad -$$
$$LI - KI$$

Functions:

1) Regulates Circulation of Qi and Blood through the Lower Jiao.

2) Calms the Shen.

3) Supplements Yin.

4) Harmonizes the Intestines.

Primary Complaints: Headaches, IBS, insomnia, liver disease, palpitations, anemia, costal pain, stress.

2nd or 3rd Concerns: Constipation, abdominal pain, colitis, low back pain, kidney disease, infertility, amenorrhea, low libido.

Explanation:

This circuit is often used when stress or chronic emotional repression has injured the jue yin, and has been compounded with overwork, adrenal burnout, excessive sex, drug abuse, or other activities that deplete the kidneys. It is particularly useful for liver and kidney yin deficiency patterns. Since the kidney water is the mother of liver wood, and the blood and essence share the same source, this circuit has wide applications for these types of patterns.

This circuit is especially effective when liver and kidney patterns combine and occur with symptoms such as constipation, shen disturbance, fatigue, anemia, infertility, and gynecological disorders. It is also very good for various conditions of the lower abdominal and chest that are due to liver imbalances.

This circuit is important to consider when patients present with chest and abdominal symptoms and a pre-dominance of liver and kidney patterns. The Yin Wei and Yin Qiao both strongly influence the chest and abdomen and are important for many reasons. While the PC meridian links the LV and KI channels, PC 6 functions to open the chest, resolve stagnations, and harmonize the stomach. Since PC 6 also opens the Yin Wei, which nourishes the yin and blood, it plays an important adjunct role in cases of liver and kidney yin deficiency. It should also be recalled that the Yin Wei starts at KI 9, and has a crossing point at LV 14, this makes the use of PC 6 very important for conditions that simultaneously manifest liver and kidney patterns.

The Yin Qiao is opened by KI 6 and may be used to treat abdominal distress when constipation is present. Since KI 6 is one of the best points to supplement the kidney yin it is useful for constipation due to yin or blood deficiency. Kidney 6 is also well known for calming the shen, opening the chest, and promoting the functions of the uterus. This makes the combination of KI 6 and PC 6 very effective for chest and abdominal conditions that are caused by liver disharmony, and present with kidney yin deficient signs.

Metal Overacts on Wood and Nourishes Water

The presence of the LI in this circuit is very effective for patterns that present with low back pain and liver stagnation. While it is commonly known that LI 4 resolves liver qi stagnation, it is also the source point and therefore connects to the kidney. Related to the functions of LI 4, but with a more powerful effect, the point Ling Ku is able to effectively resolve low back pain. Ling Ku (LK) is best combined with Da Bai (DB), and both of these points are located on the LI meridian; they are indispensable for treating low back pain and liver qi stagnation simultaneously. In addition, Dr. Wei-Chieh Young states that LK benefits the qi, warms the yang, and effects the kidneys, and this is one reason it is so effective for lumbar pain and sciatica.

From a 5-element perspective metal is able to control wood and benefit water. Therefore, LK, DB, and LI 4 are useful for conditions of liver disharmony occurring with kidney deficiency.

This circuit also has broad applications in the treatment of many gynecological diseases that present with liver and kidney patterns. The use of the LI and LV meridians are very effective for resolving stagnations; and the PC channel treats stagnation of qi and blood, strongly influences the abdomen, and nourishes both yin and blood through the Yin Wei. The KI meridian supplements and treats imbalances in the kidneys, and provides the foundational support for gynecological conditions with kidney deficiency. This circuit may be used for PMS, amenorrhea, menopause, infertility, and difficult menstruation.

CHAPTER 7

INTERNAL-EXTERNAL CIRCUITS

There are a three more 4M circuits that we have not yet covered that are most appropriately grouped according to their internal/external relationships. For example, the lungs and large intestine are connected through system three and may form a 4M circuit with the kidney and urinary bladder. Likewise the HT, SI, LV, and GB also form a 4M circuit, as do the ST, SP, SJ, and PC. These circuits are represented below.

HT - SI	SP - ST	KI - UB
- -	- -	- -
GB - LV	SJ - PC	LI - LU

These circuits are of particular interest from a 5-element perspective because of the way they pair adjacent elements. In the circuit that contains the KI, UB, LU, and LI, we find that both metal and water are represented; we therefore refer to this circuit as the metal-water circuit. In the wood-fire circuit we find the HT, SI, LV, and GB, while in the earth-fire circuit the SP, ST, SJ, and PC are present.

As we discuss these circuits we will not distinguish between primary and secondary concerns as we have done for the previous ones. This is because any circuit that contains the same four meridians ultimately has the same functions, and by now the reader should be familiar enough with the reasons for asking about the patient's top three health concerns. This is done for the purpose of prioritizing their health needs, as well as assisting the therapist in determining root patterns of disharmony. So rather than repeating ourselves by explaining the inverse circuits, the reader should take it upon themselves to determine how the patient's priorities and root patterns pertain to what they encounter in clinic.

METAL – WATER CIRCUIT

LU - LI

-      -

UB - KI

Functions:

1) Governs Respiration and Excretion.

2) Regulates Water Metabolism.

3) Harmonizes the Lower Jiao.

4) Benefits the Wei Qi.

Indications: Low back pain, colitis, constipation, asthma, infertility, incontinence, frequent urination, impotence, infertility, psoriasis.

Explanation:

This is a very important circuit for various symptoms involving the lower jiao. The kidneys, bladder, and large intestine are all located in the lower jiao, and the lung meridian crosses through here due to its connection to the LI and RN meridians. This circuit is also helpful for various respiratory conditions that are rooted in lung and kidney patterns.

This circuit is commonly used for low back pain, and it accounts for many of the ways in which this condition may be approached. Ling Ku and Da Bai are both located on the LI meridian and are extremely powerful for treating lumbar pain and sciatica. In many cases it is better to choose these points over local points on the UB channel; this is especially true for acute conditions as well as chronic lumbar pain that manifests with very tight muscles. For chronic conditions palpation should be done on the local area to assess the relative tautness of the muscles. If the tension is visible by observing the muscle tone, or if the points are very reactive to even light touch, it is often best to treat the pain by needling Ling Ku and Da Bai, along with one or two other points on the hand that are indicated for lumbar pain. These may include Yao Tong Xue, SI 3, or SI 4. The points should be needled on the opposite side of the pain.

For low back pain along the UB meridian, adding LU 5 and nearby ashi points can be especially effective. This is because the LU and UB meridians share system two and four correspondences, the elbow images the lumbar area, and metal generates water in the 5-element cycle. For these reasons the lung meridian can benefit the kidneys. In particular, LU 5 is useful for lumbar pain, descending fluids to the bladder, and is the water point on the metal meridian; it is therefore very helpful for benefiting the water energies.

WOOD – FIRE CIRCUIT

HT - SI

\-   \-

GB - LV

Functions:

1) Governs Circulation of Qi and Blood.

2) Calms the Shen.

3) Clears Heat.

4) Benefits Heart and Liver Functions.

Indications: Hypertension, stress, palpitations, neck and shoulder tension, liver and gallbladder channel headaches, shen disturbance, liver disease, enteritis, and hepatitis.

Explanation:

This is a powerful circuit that governs circulation of qi and blood and is especially important for liver and heart imbalances. In terms of 5-elements, this circuit is used when there are imbalances in the wood and fire energies and symptoms exist in the HT, SI, LV, or GB channels. Since wood generates fire in the 5-element cycle, we often find that liver imbalances can effect the heart in adverse ways. This can be seen in cases where liver fire leads to heart fire, and the way in which liver yang is associated with hypertension. When liver imbalances effect the heart, it is good to use points on the GB channel since the GB connects to both the liver and heart meridians.

This circuit is also very useful for treating neck and shoulder tension along the SI and GB meridians, especially when there is an underlying liver imbalance. It is common for liver qi stagnation to affect the neck, upper back, shoulders, jaw, and head, and when symptoms present along the GB and SI channels in these areas, this circuit is often a good choice. When an underlying liver pattern also presents with shen disturbance, the use of heart points to calm the mind are an important part of the overall treatment strategy.

This circuit is ideal for someone that has a type A personality with symptoms such as shen disturbance, heart disease, hypertension, liver imbalance, neck, shoulder, and upper back pain.

EARTH - FIRE CIRCUIT

SP - ST
- -
SJ - PC

Functions:

1) Benefits and Harmonizes Digestion.

2) Supplements Qi and Blood.

3) Clears Heat, Resolves Damp.

4) Calms the Shen, Benefits Blood and Yin.

Indications: Weak digestion, low appetite, fatigue, acid reflux, diarrhea, constipation, stomach ulcers, gastritis, heat sensations, headaches, heart diseases related to blood deficiency or blood stagnation.

Explanation:

This is a fundamental fire-earth circuit that is important for conditions of the digestive system, in which there is either an excess of heat or a deficiency of yang qi. When excessive heat or fire is present in the stomach it can be regulated and cleared through the fire meridians of the pericardium and san jiao. The pericardium points PC 3 and PC 6 are well known for their ability to regulate the stomach and abdomen, and they may serve to drain excess heat or fire from the stomach as well. The san jiao has a connection to the spleen, and is well known for clearing heat and resolving dampness. For this reason, this circuit can also be used for spleen damp heat patterns.

From a 5-element perspective the pericardium and san jiao meridians are a good choice for supplementing spleen qi and yang deficiency. This is because strengthening the fire helps to supplement the earth element. For this type of treatment strategy the PC meridian is a better choice than the HT meridian, since the PC has a direct link to the stomach and spleen. Numerous points on the PC meridian are indicated for stomach and abdominal conditions, and the coupling of PC 6 and SP 4 helps to boost the spleen function. Though the heart meridian has a direct connection to the spleen through system five, we do not find indications on the HT meridian for stomach and abdominal conditions like we do on the PC meridian.

Although the san jiao is not typically used for boosting yang, it may be used to supplement the fire and yang through the use of moxa. Remember that the san jiao shares a system four association with the spleen, a system two connection to the kidneys, and functions to transport yaun qi to the middle jiao. For these reasons, as well as the 5-element associations, we can use the SJ meridian to boost spleen qi and yang.

CHAPTER 8

REFLECTIONS ON THE PATTERNS

The preceding chapters introduced a total of 15 unique meridian circuits, and these form the basis of doing pattern identification that is derived from the connections between the channels. Each of these 15 circuits may therefore be spoken of as a syndrome, and it is possible to do syndrome differentiation using only these circuits. For instance, we may speak of a yang ming - jue yin pattern, and this syndrome would consist of characteristic symptoms such as constipation, ulcers, acid reflux, headaches, palpitations, anemia, and tightness in the chest and hypochondrium. We may also speak of the yang ming - tai yin syndrome as being characterized by digestive and respiratory symptoms. The shao yin - shao yang pattern is defined by symptoms such as palpitations, low back pain, temple or occipital headaches, muscle twitches, tinnitus, insomnia, and shen disturbance.

To do syndrome differentiation based on the connections between the meridians, it is essential to learn the five meridian systems, as well as the characteristic signs and symptoms for the each of the 4M circuits. While it is possible, and in some cases even beneficial, to do pattern identification using only the five meridian systems and 15 circuits, it is often appropriate to combine circuit differentiation with zang-fu diagnostic methods. As an example, let's examine a case with a primary complaint of headaches, a secondary concern of palpitations, and he suffers from constipation as well. This person also has stomach ulcers and acid reflux. Using the meridian systems and 4M circuit differentiation, we find that the jue yin - yang ming circuit is able to address all of the patient's concerns. However, it is also helpful to determine what zang-fu patterns are present. In the above situation the patient's root cause could be liver qi stagnation, liver fire, yin deficiency, blood deficiency, or any number of other patterns. By identifying circuit patterns, and zang-fu syndromes, the therapist is able to more accurately diagnose root patterns of disharmony.

Similarly, if one has identified a root pattern of liver fire, it is essential to determine what organs or meridians are most adversely effected. Since liver fire may effect the pericardium, heart, gallbladder, stomach, lungs, and large intestine; clearly identifying what organs are most effected by the liver fire, is essential to refining our treatment strategies and point selections. If the fire is mostly effecting the heart, stomach, and large intestine, then it is most appropriate to use the jue yin - yang ming circuit, as opposed to using a circuit that contains the gallbladder and lung meridans.

To accurately determine what 4M circuit is primarily responsible for the patient's symptoms, it is essential to ask about the client's top three health concerns. This allows the therapist to more clearly identify the *primary* 4M circuit that is in disharmony, and also assists in determining what zang-fu pattern is most problematic. By using the technique of asking the patient about their top three health concerns, with 4M circuit and zang-fu pattern identification methods, the therapist is able to develop highly refined diagnostic skills and treatment strategies.

While the 4M circuits are fundamental to doing meridian based pattern identification, it may not always be possible to associate a client's priorities and patterns to one particular 4M circuit. In these cases it may be necessary to add one or two meridians to a circuit, to account for their chief symptoms and root patterns of imbalance. Though we have already introduced how to add meridians to the circuits, we shall continue to build on this concept through this chapter. To begin, let's examine an actual case study where dampness was the main pathogenic factor.

CASE STUDY: Female, 46

Primary Complaint: Right knee pain and swelling along the SP meridian. The pain was located at SP 9 and the whole medial portion of the knee was visibly swollen. With palpation the SP meridian was sensitive and in particular SP 9 was most reactive. The patient also had a cyst at UB 40, and had one removed from the same location two years prior to coming in for acupuncture.

Secondary Concern: Left sided neck pain located near SJ 16 and extending through the SJ meridian. The pain would also radiate into the GB and UB meridians when severe.

Third Concern: IBS with loose stool, bloating, tiredness, and water retention.

The tongue was pale and puffy with teeth marks.

The accumulation of dampness involving the SP meridian in the region of knee was very apparent with observation. Internally, the spleen organ was also severely effected by the dampness, and this manifested with typical spleen damp symptoms. To treat the main concern of knee pain and swelling in the SP and UB channels, it is optimum to use the LU meridian, since it connects to both the SP and UB.

To address the underlying damp pattern that was rooted in a SP imbalance, the SP and ST pair should also be used in the overall treatment strategy. This means that the 4M circuit that is most appropriate for treating this patient is the tai yin - yang ming circuit. Notice how the LI meridian's inclusion in this circuit also addresses the IBS.

SP - LU
- -
ST - LI

As complete as this circuit is for addressing the client's primary and tertiary concerns, it does not account for the secondary concern of neck pain. When palpation was done, there was a large muscle knot located precisely at SJ 16, when pressed it caused radiating sensations to SJ 17 and GB 20. To address this condition it was decided to add the SJ meridian to the treatment strategy. This was done not only for the neck pain, but also because the SJ plays an important role in water metabolism and can help to resolve damp accumulation. Taking all this into consideration we can construct the following circuit.

SJ - SP - LU
- -
ST - LI

The points used for treatment were: right side LU 5, LU 7, ST 36, ST 40; left side SP 3, SP 9, SJ 5, LI 11.

As mentioned the LU meridian can address conditions with both the SP and UB meridians, and is therefore the most important meridian for resolving the primary complaint. While LU 5 mirrors the knee, it also functions energetically to resolve dampness; LU 7 was added because it is the luo point, and greatly effects the LI and nape of the neck, it is therefore helpful for addressing both the secondary and tertiary concerns. The stomach points help to strengthen the SP, and resolve damp and phlegm, while LI 11 resolves dampness from the colon. On the spleen meridian SP 3 was used because it resolves dampness, images the neck, and shares a system four connection with the SJ. The final point SJ 5 treats neck pain and assists in resolving dampness. Although there was swelling and a cyst located at UB 40 on the knee, the UB meridian was not needled.

The above case demonstrates one example of how to easily incorporate a meridian into a 4M circuit; however, to do this effectively there are a few things that need to be considered. First of all, when using meridian systems methodologies it is most beneficial to identify a 4M circuit. A fifth meridian should only be added when it is warranted by a symptomatic expression in the meridian, or when the meridian will have a direct effect on the organ that is most out of balance. For the above case the most appropriate zang-fu pattern would be classified as spleen damp obstruction. Since the SJ directly connects to the SP, and is manifesting a secondary symptom, it is necessary to add it to our treatment protocol.

Another important point to consider when adding an extra meridian to a 4M circuit, is that it is possible to connect any of the channels through either one or two meridians. For example, the SJ and LU are not directly connected, but they both connect to the SP. This can be represented as:

LU - SP - SJ

If we follow this line of reasoning to all the meridians, we will find that no channels are separated by more than 2 places. For instance, the GB and UB represent two meridians that are not directly connected, but they often have simultaneous symptoms, especially in cases of sciatica. To connect these meridians we have to go through the LV and SI, the HT and KI, or the SJ and KI. These connections are represented as:

GB - LV - SI - UB

GB - HT - KI - UB

GB - SJ - KI - UB

From these associations we can construct various circuits, and the circuit used will depend on the patient's chief concerns and overall pattern. For patterns of sciatica that occur with liver or lung symptoms, or are due to qi and blood stagnation, we may choose to work with the tai yang – LV/LU circuit.

UB - SI
-        -
LU - LV - GB

If a sciatic pattern presents with kidney deficiency, heart imbalance, or disharmony between the heart and kidney, we could use the tai yang - shao yin circuit.

UB - SI
-     -
KI - HT - GB

Alternately, if a patient complains of sciatica due to kidney deficiency, and they also have spleen qi and heart blood deficiency, we could use the following circuit.

UB - KI - HT - GB
-     -
SJ - SP

When we start adding meridians to the 4M circuits we end up with modified circuits that are able to account for complex cases that manifest with multiple patterns. In cases like this it is essential to identify the most pertinent 4M circuit that is out of balance, and then develop a treatment strategy based around that circuit. After this has been done, one or two meridians may be added to the circuit to give maximum results by accounting for the numerous patterns that are present. To understand how this works, let's compare two examples of sciatica that occur with different secondary and tertiary complaints.

In the first case the patient is a 33 year-old man with a primary complaint of left-sided sciatica in the UB and GB channels. Secondarily he suffers from chronic diarrhea with undigested food, and his third concern is asthma with profuse watery phlegm. According to zang-fu pattern identification he suffers from kidney deficiency, and this contributes to both the diarrhea and asthma. As a final analysis we conclude that he has a kidney yang deficiency, causing spleen and lung yang vacuities.

Based on the underlying kidney yang deficiency, we decide to address his primary concern of sciatica in the UB and GB channels with the UB - KI pair. To begin to construct a

4M circuit we start with:

UB - KI

Since the GB does not directly connect to either of these meridians, we decide to continue our construction of the circuit based on his secondary and tertiary complaints. Knowing that the UB connects to the LU, and the LU connects to the SP, we arrive at the following:

UB - KI

-

LU

-

SP

To finish the circuit we find that the LI connects to both the KI and LU, and this allows us to complete the Metal - Water circuit.

UB - KI

-    -

LU - LI

-

SP

Notice that the LI meridian naturally fits into the circuit, and most importantly, it plays a major role in addressing his primary, secondary and tertiary complaints. The two points Ling Ku and Da Bai, located on the LI meridian, are indicated for sciatica in the tai yang and shao yang channels. In addition, these two points also supplement and warm the yang, and treat respiratory diseases. Therefore, these two points are capable of addressing all of the branch symptoms, while treating the underlying root pattern of kidney yang deficiency. This can also be understood in 5-element terms because metal engenders water. It is through methods like this that one can develop the capacity to treat numerous symptoms and complex patterns with only a few needles.

Since the patient has a secondary concern related to the SP function, we decide to use points on the SP meridian such as SP 3, and this point also benefits the spine. Spleen 9 can also be added because it transforms damp, and treats problems due to spleen and kidney deficiencies. Alternately, we may replace SP 9 with Shen Guan (77.18), which is located 1.5 cun below SP 9. This point's name translates as Kidney Gate, and it is useful for treating sciatica, lumbar pain, and has the function of benefiting both the spleen and kidneys.

To address the tertiary complaint of asthma we want to be aware of a few dynamics that are going on within the patient. First, we know that the root pattern is based in a kidney deficiency, so we want to choose points that will have a mutual benefit on the kidneys and lungs. We may also want to use the 5-element method of boosting the earth to engender metal, since his secondary concern is related to the earth element and the spleen. To account for these patterns lets return our attention to the circuit.

UB - KI

\-   -

SP - LU - LI

We may recall that there are many ST points that are indicated for asthma and these include: ST 36, ST 40, and most notably 88.17, 88.18, and 88.19. We can now add the ST meridian to the above circuit.

147

UB - KI
-     -
LU - LI
-     -
SP - ST

By adding the SP and ST meridians to the Metal - Water circuit, we are able to account for the patient's secondary concern, and utilize 5-element methods to address his third concern of asthma.

In conclusion we arrive at the following point prescription: right side Ling Ku, Da Bai, KI 7, Shen Guan; left side LU 5, LU 9, ST 36, ST 40, or replace ST 36 and ST 40 with 88.17, 88.18, 88.19.

Notice that the GB meridian was not added to our circuit even though the meridian was symptomatic. This channel was excluded because it did not fit within the most logical circuit to use when we account for his main concerns and underlying zang-fu pattern.

Case 2

Let's now take a look at another case who is a 52 year-old man that suffers from sciatica on the left side. Like the first client the pain is present in the UB and GB channels, but he also complains of upper back pain along the SI meridian in the region of SI 11 and SI 13. Secondarily he suffers from temple headaches in the GB meridian, and they are worse with stress and overwork. His final concern is a history of hepatitis. Without going into all the other signs and symptoms present, it was concluded that he suffers from kidney yin deficiency and liver fire. Listing his main complaints with the imbalanced meridians and organs looks as such.

Primary Concern: Sciatica - UB and GB; Upper back pain - UB and SI

Secondary Concern: Temple Headaches - GB

Tertiary Concern: Hepatitis - LV

Taking all this into consideration we know that the UB and GB are primary meridians to work with. However, there is no direct connection between them, so we need to consider what meridians will connect them while addressing his root patterns.

Since he also has pain in the SI meridian, and this was a part of his primary concern, we decide to start with the tai yang pair.

UB - SI

Since the primary concern of sciatica is rooted in a kidney deficiency, we decide to add the KI to our developing circuit.

UB - SI
-
KI

It should also be noticed that the HT meridian may be added since it connects to both the SI and KI, and this would leave us with the tai yang - shao yin circuit.

UB - SI
-   -
KI - HT

To address the GB meridian sciatica and temple headaches we can also add the shao yang pair to our circuit.

UB - SI
-      -
KI - HT
-      -
SJ - GB

While this circuit could be used, the presence of the heart meridian doesn't best serve the overall pattern that is present. So even though we have a circuit that connects the UB and GB, and addresses the kidney deficiency, it doesn't adequately account for the presence of liver fire. Reviewing our meridian connections and looking for a replacement for the HT meridian, we find that the LV connects to both the SI and GB. This leads us to the following circuit.

UB - SI
-      -
KI   LV
-      -
SJ - GB

Although there is no direct connection between the KI and LV in meridian systems theory, the presence of the liver in the circuit fits better with the patient's overall presentation than the HT channel does. For this reason this is the main circuit we would use to treat this case.

As a final note on the above circuit notice how SJ points can address the sciatica, temple headaches, hepatitis, and liver fire. The SI can treat sciatica and upper back pain, and the SI channel can also treat hepatitis through the use of SI 4, 33.10, and 33.11.

Analysis

Comparing these two cases we find that both of them had a primary concern of sciatica in the UB and GB channels; however, through inquiring about their top three concerns we were able to account for their zang-fu patterns and make more intelligent point prescriptions. In summary, when the method of inquiring about their health priorities is combined with meridian systems theory, it can guide us in determining zang-fu patterns, and designing highly effective treatment strategies.

Circuits with 6 Meridians

Before completing this chapter a few final words on 6M circuits is necessary. As shown above, using circuits with 6 meridians can be extremely beneficial for unraveling complex cases, but 6M circuits should only be used when absolutely necessary. If the case can be treated with a 4M circuit, rather than a 6M circuit, it is often best to limit the meridians used to only those that are most crucial to the treatment. Using too many meridians and points can dilute the results, lead to poor point combinations, and is a sign that inaccurate pattern identification is occurring. However, when meridian systems theory is used in conjunction with zang-fu methodologies, it can greatly assist in making more accurate diagnoses and treatment strategies. In the following chapter we will continue to build on how meridian systems and circuit theory integrates with zang-fu patterns.

CHAPTER 9

CIRCUIT THEORY AND ZANG-FU METHODS OF PATTERN IDENTIFICATION

This chapter will cover two common conditions that are encountered in clinic that respond very will to acupuncture therapy. In each section we will review the classical TCM patterns, and then demonstrate how circuit theory may be applied to each of the associated syndromes. Let's begin by covering headaches.

Headaches

When we compare traditional methods of diagnosing headaches with meridian systems and circuit theory, we find many interesting points of overlap. In conventional teachings there are two major methods used to arrive at pattern identification for headaches, the first is based on the location of the pain according to the channels, and the second one utilizes internal organ patterns of disharmony. These two methods are often used together and help to refine the diagnostic process. For example, when headaches are located at the top of the head they are usually identified as a jue yin pattern, and may be caused by either liver yang rising or liver blood deficiency. In contrast, headaches located at the forehead are typically regarded as

152

a yang ming pattern and may be due to stomach heat, dampness, or phlegm. A typical approach to diagnosing headaches is to first determine the location of the pain according to channel theory, and then follow with zang-fu diagnostic methodologies to determine the internal organ pattern.

When using the meridian systems and 4M circuits in pattern identification and treatment, we should determine what circuit is most out of balance according to the patient chief symptoms. This is done according to the methodologies already described, and includes identifying what locations in the head are affected, and asking the patient about their top three health concerns. After this the meridian systems are used to identify the appropriate circuit for treatment. Like conventional methods we may also integrate our understanding of internal organ patterns into our diagnosis, and this can help us to determine what circuit is primarily out of balance.

The following sections show how the various 4M circuits overlap with zang-fu patterns, and how these two methods of diagnose may be used together. Though this is a simplified approach it can be insightful to make these comparisons. In the following tables the circuits are located on the left side, and the various zang-fu patterns that may be treated with the circuits are listed on the right side.

Shao Yang Headaches and Associated Patterns

Shao Yang – Jue Yin	Liver yang, liver fire, liver wind, liver qi stagnation.
Shao Yang – Shao Yin	Kidney, essence, blood, and qi deficiency patterns.
Shao Yang – Spleen/Heart	Liver wind, stasis of blood, blood and qi deficiency, dampness.

The temples and side of the head are associated with the shao yang, and more specifically the GB. Headaches located here are typically associated with liver yang, liver fire, and liver wind. In cases where the underlying pattern is rooted in a liver syndrome, it is best to use the shao yang – jue yin circuit, as this is the most commonly used circuit for shao yang headaches. However, since the shao yang also connects to the shao yin, and the heart and spleen, we need to be aware of other internal organ imbalances that can be causative factors. If a spleen qi and heart blood deficiency pattern is present, it can cause headaches in the temples due to the link between the heart and gallbladder, and blood deficiency and wind. Similarly, kidney deficiency may also be connected to temple headaches, since a deficiency of the kidneys can lead to liver yang rising and liver wind.

Yang Ming Headaches and Associated Patterns

Yang Ming – Jue Yin	Stomach heat, retention of food, turbid phlegm, liver qi stagnation, blood deficiency.
Yang Ming – Tai Yin	Qi deficiency, blood deficiency, stomach heat, food retention, blood stasis, turbid phlegm, dampness.
Yang Ming – KI/PC	Kidney deficiency, blood deficiency, qi deficiency, stomach heat, blood stasis, retention of food, dampness.

Frontal headaches are often due to damp or phlegm in the head, and this prevents the clear yang from ascending. If the kidneys, spleen, or lungs are deficient, this can cause excess water or phlegm to build in the body and cause frontal headaches. In these cases it is essential to treat the root cause of the build up of pathogenic fluids.

Since the yang ming is said to contain abundant qi and blood, qi and blood deficiency patterns may also be an underlying cause of yang ming pattern headaches. In these cases there is often a deficiency in the spleen's ability to produce blood from the food and nutrients. Likewise, liver or heart/pericardium blood deficiency, may also contribute to frontal headaches, and this can be treated with the yang ming - jue yin circuit.

Tai Yang Headaches

Tai Yang – Tai Yin	Wind cold, wind heat, wind damp, damp, turbid phlegm, blood stasis, qi deficiency, blood deficiency
Tai Yang – Shao Yin	Kidney deficiency, qi deficiency, blood deficiency, blood stasis
Tai Yang – LU/LV	External invasions, liver wind, liver qi stagnation, cold in the liver channel, damp, blood stasis, qi deficiency

In traditional theories tai yang headaches are most often associated with kidney deficiency and external invasions. For externally caused conditions, the tai yang - tai yin circuit is most often used, and this is because the tai yin includes the lung meridian. The tai yang - tai yin circuit is also effective when secondary concerns relate to spleen or lung deficiencies. Similarly, spleen qi vacuity can cause blood deficiency or damp accumulation, and both of these patterns may be connected to tai yang headaches.

For cases where kidney deficiency is the underlying cause, the tai yang - shao yin circuit is clearly preferable. Essence and blood vacuity patterns may be treated with the tai yang - shao yin circuit, since the kidneys store the essence, and the heart has a strong association with blood production and circulation. For tai yang headaches with an underlying blood deficiency, the shao yin is also useful because "the blood and essence share the same source."

Jue Yin Headaches

Jue yin headaches are generally thought of as affecting the top of the head or the eyes. This is because the liver meridian extends to the vertex, and the eyes are related to the liver. The circuits that are formed with the jue yin are as follows.

Jue Yin – Yang Ming	Liver qi stagnation, liver fire, turbid phlegm, wind phlegm, blood stasis, retention of food, stomach heat, qi deficiency, blood deficiency
Jue Yin – Shao Yang	Liver yang, liver fire, liver wind, liver qi stagnation, dampness, phlegm, wind phlegm, blood stasis
Jue Yin – LI/KI	Liver yang, liver wind, liver qi stagnation, dampness, blood stasis, qi deficiency, blood deficiency, kidney deficiency

The jue yin - yang ming circuit works very well for headaches that occur behind the eyes and in the forehead. It is ideal for treating liver qi stagnation patterns, blood stasis, stomach patterns, and phlegm. Since both the stomach and pericardium meridians are able to resolve turbid phlegm, this circuit is ideal for cases that manifest with phlegm signs in the upper jiao, stomach, and head.

In cases of jue yin pattern headaches due to kidney deficiency, or liver yang rising, the jue yin - LI/KI circuit may be used. While the large intestine meridian helps to resolve liver imbalance, it also serves to nourish the kidney by way of the 5-element cycle. When used for this purpose, it is best to use Ling Ku because it has a strong effect on moving liver qi and supplementing the kidneys.

Temple Headaches and Liver Patterns

The shao yang - jue yin circuit should be used when the primary complaint is temple headaches along the GB channel, and secondary concerns or zang-fu patterns indicate an imbalance in the liver. Liver disharmonies that may be treated with this circuit include liver qi stagnation, liver fire, liver yang rising, or liver wind. If the secondary or tertiary concerns involve symptoms that affect the GB, SJ, LV, or PC, this circuit will usually be sufficient for the treatment. However, in certain cases the underlying internal organ pattern may effect other meridians and systems that are not included in this circuit. For example, let's take a look at a patient who has a primary concern of temple headaches, a secondary concern of abdominal pain, and a tertiary complaint of constipation. The pulse is wiry and the tongue is slightly red on the sides. The patient also lives a fast paced and stressful lifestyle. Taking all the signs and symptoms into consideration, the pattern is identified as liver qi stagnation, with insufficient evidence of any liver fire or heat signs.

Since the primary concern is headaches in the temple and GB channel, with underlying liver qi stagnation, we decide to use the shao yang - jue yin circuit. However, the secondary and tertiary complaints involve the abdomen and large intestine, and therefore point to an imbalance in the yang ming. Taking all this in to consideration we arrive at the need to use the following 6M circuit.

158

Primary Symptoms Affect	GB - SJ	Temple Headaches
	- -	
Root Pattern Involves	LV - PC	Liver Qi Stagnation
	- -	
2nd and 3rd Concerns	LI - ST	Pain, Constipation

Since we are trying to maximize our results with the fewest needles possible, we need to pay particular attention to the yang meridians. For both the foot and hand yang meridians we have two pairs to work with. On the hand we need to choose points on the LI and SJ meridians, and on the leg the ST and GB channels are represented. The primary concern is headaches, so we should put some priority on the GB and SJ meridians, as well as points that can best resolve the headaches. In the case of the SJ meridian, SJ 3 or SJ 5 are good choices as they are both indicated for headaches, while SJ 6 is indicated for the third concern of constipation. Since the condition is rooted in a liver qi stagnation pattern, we would also be wise to chose LI 4 or Ling Ku, as both of these points soothe liver qi, stop headaches, and are useful in abdominal complaints.

On the leg we need to work with both the GB and ST channels, and we want to select the points that will give us the greatest benefits. In the case of the GB channel we will use the technique of imaging the head to the feet and confine our selections to GB points on the foot. Many GB points are indicated for headaches such as GB 41, GB 42, GB 43, and GB 44; but we also want to keep the patient's secondary complaints in mind, even though there is no direct connection between the GB and yang ming. Knowing that GB 41 opens the Dai, and influences the abdomen, it would be best to choose this point out of all our available choices. In regards to our final point selection on the ST channel, we should begin by palpating the ST meridian from ST 36 – ST 37. We should also check for reactive points between the GB and ST channels between

ST 36 and GB 34.

The points selected on the yin meridians are much easier to choose since we only have to select from the LV and PC channels. On the PC meridian needle PC 3 and PC 6, and on the LV channel LV 3 should be selected as well as the most reactive point between LV 7 and LV 8.

Our final point selection is: right side PC 3, PC 6, GB 41, ST 36 or ST 37 or the most reactive point between the ST and GB channels; left side points include SJ 3, SJ 5, LK, LV 3, LV 7 or LV 8.

The above example demonstrates how circuit theory integrates with zang-fu pattern diagnosis, but allows one to more effectively make point selections based on root conditions and the patient's priorities. When meridian systems and the client's chief concerns are taken into consideration, with zang-fu methods of syndrome differentiation, greater precision can be made when making point selections. One of the greatest strengths of circuit theory is to simplify complex patterns and effectively make point selections that give the greatest synergy and clinical results.

Dysmenorrhea

Painful periods are a very common condition encountered in clinic and respond very well to acupuncture therapy. While traditional methods of syndrome differentiation recognize several patterns of imbalance, meridian systems and circuit theory is able to utilize numerous circuits based on the patient's predominate symptoms. The major meridian pairs used in circuit theory for the treatment of dysmenorrhea are the jue yin, yang ming, and tai yin. In liver related patterns it is usually most appropriate to use the jue yin - yang ming circuit, while in patterns that manifest with more spleen, damp, or cold signs, it is often best to use the tai yin - yang ming circuit. Though there are other circuits that may be used to treat dysmenorrhea, the jue yin - yang ming, and tai yin - yang ming circuits will be sufficient to cover most cases. Before we discuss the circuits any further lets quickly review traditional patterns recognized in the treatment of this disease. They are:

1. Stagnation of Qi and Blood
2. Stagnation of Cold
3. Stagnation of Damp Heat
4. Qi and Blood Deficiency
5. Kidney and Liver Deficiency

Qi and Blood Stagnation

Since this is one of the most common patterns let's discuss how the circuits may be used for treating this pattern. As usual the circuit used depends on the patient's top health concerns and overall presentations.

In the first case the patient's chief concern is painful periods. When asked more precisely about the symptoms she complains of abdominal distension that is located

161

diffusely throughout her lower abdomen. The pain starts one or two days before menstruation and continues until day two or three. The pain is severe and is not localized or fixed in a precise location, but she does have clots for the first two days. During her period she has headaches that are located across the forehead, and she also has water retention with minor swelling around the ankles. The period lasts for five days. Her secondary concern is abdominal pain that seems to be connected to her diet, although she has not been able to discern what foods cause it; but she does know that the pain is worse when she is hungry. Her third health concern is poor immunity, and she gets sick with common colds about three times a year. Her tongue is slightly puffy and the pulse is rolling and choppy.

The above case could be identified as a qi and blood stagnation pattern since she has pain, headaches, clots, and a choppy pulse. Typical points for qi and blood stagnation patterns include: LI 4, LV 3, GB 34, RN 6, ST 29, SP 10, SP 8, SP 6, LU 7, KI 6, SP 4, and PC 6. Though it is not ideal to needle all these points at the same time, these are the most common points indicated for painful periods due to qi and blood stagnation.

When we approach the above case with circuit theory methodologies, we are looking for the circuit that is most out of balance. In this case we find that spleen symptoms predominate over liver symptoms. The spleen symptoms are seen in the quality of the abdominal pain, the presence of yang ming headaches, as well as in the water retention and ankle swelling. Her tongue and pulse signs also indicate an imbalance in the spleen, and the third concern of low immunity confirms that the tai yin and lungs are involved.

Though we could properly identify the above case as a qi and blood stagnation pattern, we should pay careful attention to the lack of liver signs and symptoms. In cases of qi and blood stagnation, it is common to arrive at the conclusion that liver qi stagnation is the causative factor; however, in many cases there is actually a predominance of spleen imbalances. The above case demonstrates this, and shows why it is important to distinguish between using the tai yin - yang ming circuit, and the jue yin - yang ming circuit.

The tai yin - yang ming circuit is used for qi and blood stagnation patterns, when there is a predominance of tai yin symptoms. When this circuit is used LI points like LI 4, Ling Ku, 33.10, 33.02, and 33.03 are used to resolve the qi stagnation; and SP points like SP 4, SP 6, SP 8, and SP 10 are used to regulate and move the blood. For the above case a final point prescription using the tai yin - yang ming circuit is left side: SP 4, SP 9, SP 10, LI 4, LK; and right side LU 5, LU 7, ST 36.

Let's now examine another case that has similar but slightly different signs and symptoms. This patient's chief concern is painful periods that are so intense that she needs to take time off from work. When asked about accompanying symptoms she complains of headaches that start in the middle of her head and then go into her eyes. She also gets low back pain during menstruation, and she frequently feels this at other times as well. There are no clots in the menstrual blood and the period lasts for 4 days. Her secondary complaint is insomnia that she has suffered from for many years. Her third concern is low back pain, it is worse on the right side, and there is no history of an injury that she can remember. Her tongue is slightly red with some small cracks in the center. Her pulse is thin and choppy.

This case demonstrates how numerous syndromes may be present, and can lead to complexities when trying to identify traditional zang-fu patterns. Liver qi stagnation can be seen in the quality of the pain, as well as in the headaches that effect the eyes. Blood stagnation signs are present even in the absence of menstrual clots, and they can be seen in the severity of the pain, as well as in the choppy pulse. Finally, we should acknowledge that the kidneys are involved since the patient has frequent low back pain, and the lumbar pain is also worse with menses. The insomnia, red tongue, and thin pulse also indicate a likely condition of kidney deficiency.

In this case it would be possible to arrive at a diagnosis of qi and blood stagnation, and/or liver and kidney deficiency. This would be an adequate assessment and numerous treatments could be designed to address these imbalances. For comparison let's see how circuit theory allows us to proceed with the case.

Since the patient presents with severe menstrual pain that occurs with headaches affecting the eyes, we decide to work with the jue yin pair. Her secondary concern of insomnia can also be addressed with this pair, since PC points are widely used for insomnia. The choppy quality of her pulse gives us the final sign we need to conclude that we should use a meridian that can move the blood. The third concern of low back pain, and the way in which this is connected to her menstrual cycle, makes us decide to use the kidney meridian as part of the treatment. This gives us the following meridians to work with.

LV - PC
-   -
KI

Now all we need is to complete the circuit with a meridian that connects to both the KI and LV. Reviewing our five systems we find that the LI meridian connects to both of them. This leaves us with the jue yin - KI/LI circuit.

LV - PC
- -
LI - KI

If we were to base our treatment strategy on the zang-fu patterns of qi and blood stagnation, with liver and kidney deficiency, we would arrive at the treatment principle of move qi and blood, resolve stasis, stop pain, nourish yin, and benefit the kidneys. All of which can be accomplished with the jue yin - KI/LI circuit. Our final point selection for this case is right side: Da Bai, Ling Ku, KI 3, KI 9, LV 3; and left side: PC 3, PC 6, GB 41.

Though the GB meridian is not part of the circuit it should be noted that no foot yang channels are present in the circuit. For this reason, and since the Dai mai can benefit the menstruation and low back pain, it is included as part of the point prescription.

Traditional Patterns of Dysmenorrhea

Traditional methods of syndrome differentiation identify five patterns of dysmenorrhea. In meridian systems there are several circuits that are commonly used for treatment. On the next page a table is presented that shows how traditional patterns of dysmenorrhea correlate with the meridian circuit systems.

Zang Fu Pattern	Circuits
Stagnation of Qi and Blood	Jue Yin – Yang Ming Tai Yin – Yang Ming Jue Yin – Shao Yang Jue Yin – LI/KI
Stagnation of Cold	Tai Yin – Yang Ming Jue Yin – Yang Ming Jue Yin – LI/KI
Damp Heat	Jue Yin – Yang Ming Jue Yin – Shao Yang Tai Yin – Yang Ming
Qi and Blood Deficiency	Tai Yin – Yang Ming
Kidney/Liver Deficiency	Jue Yin – LI/KI

As we can see from the above table there are several patterns and circuits that may be used for treating dysmennorhea. While zang-fu patterns easily integrate with circuit theory, it is not necessarily the goal to identify both zang-fu patterns and the circuit that is most out of balance. The priority of the therapist is to get the patient the relief they want, regardless of what methods of pattern identification are used. To achieve the best possible clinical results it is imperative to choose points that will provide the greatest relief, this is where circuit theory and the method of inquiring about the patient's top three concerns excels. Through identifying 4M and 6M circuits, point selections can be minimized to only those points that will provide the greatest benefit to the patient.

CHAPTER 10

CASE STUDIES

This chapter consists of numerous case studies that demonstrate the ability of the meridian circuit systems to comprehensively understand various patterns. These are actual cases that responded well with only a few treatments, and many of these clients had chronic conditions that failed to get adequate results with other therapies, including traditional forms of acupuncture.

The following cases also demonstrate how systems theory allows the clinician to simplify overly extensive and often times bulky intakes with the patient. By focusing on the patient's top three health concerns, and then identifying meridian circuits, zang-fu patterns will often readily unveil themselves. Through these examples we shall see that a circuit based approach can often help in understanding complex etiological and pathological processes. The circuit based approach to pattern differentiation is also more objective in that it focuses on the patient's priorities, and minimizes the subjective and theoretical aspects of pattern identification. This allows the clinician to identify the most fundamental patterns of disharmony, rather than those that are most obvious or secondary to the patient's needs.

167

Case Study: Female, 37

Primary Concern: Frequent Bladder Infections - UB

Secondary Concern: Bronchitis - LU

Tertiary Concern: Candida Infections and Constipation - LI

The patient suffered from frequent urinary infections for 10 years. They always started with cloudy urination and pain at the urethra, and there was also the feeling of 'expansive' pain and heaviness. After the third day blood would appear in the urine.

In regards to her secondary concern, the bronchitis had been present her whole life, and it was common for her to have intense episodes 4-5 times per year. Symptomatically she would experience sore throats, pressure in the chest with coughing, weakness, and exhaustion. The Candida infections would flare up 1-2 times per year with itching, constipation, and thick white leucorrhea being the main symptoms. When asked which of these symptoms relating to the Candida was of greatest concern, she expressed that the constipation was most problematic.

The presence of dampness in this pattern is apparent in the symptoms of cloudy urination, feelings of heaviness, and leucorrhea; the main organ being effected by the dampness is the UB. Since the bladder condition is her primary concern, let's review what meridians the UB connects to.

UB - SI - LU - KI - LU - SI

Interesting enough we find that the UB and LU share a connection through system two and four, and the LU is the primary organ involved in the patient's secondary concern. We also know that the LI connects to the LU, and it is the LI that is primarily involved in her third concern. This allows us to build the following circuit.

UB - LU

-

LI

When we compare the LU and LI meridian connections, we find that the KI connects to both of them. This leaves us with the Metal - Water Circuit.

UB - LU

-    -

KI - LI

When this patient was asked about any history of kidney disease, she stated that her mother suffers from kidney disease; and the patient also felt that her kidneys were weak, as she would occasionally feel a dull ache in them.

Points selected include left side: KI 3, KI 6, LK, LI 11; right side: LU 5, LU 7, UB 40, and ashi points on the UB meridian 2-5 cun above UB 60.

Case Study: Female, 36

Primary concern: Constipation – LI

Secondary concern: Fatigue, worse after eating as well as in the mornings and evenings, bloating also occurs after eating – SP

Tertiary concern: Sinusitis occuring with yang ming headaches – LI and ST

With the constipation and sinusitis the LI is primarily involved, the ST meridian was also effected due to the yang ming headaches and sinus pressure in the region of ST 3. For these reasons the yang ming is the primary meridian pair to work with.

When fatigue is a concern it is always important to inquire about accompanying symptoms that relate to the patterns of fatigue. For this patient, she knew that it was worse after eating and in the mornings and evenings. She also complained of bloating after eating, and for this reason the condition was identified as a spleen pattern. This allows us to use the following meridians in the construction of a circuit.

LI - ST

-

SP

To complete the circuit we add the lungs because they are the only meridian that connects to both the LI and SP.

LI - ST

-   -

LU - SP

After adding the lung meridian to the circuit, the patient was questioned about any history of lung conditions, she then revealed that she has suffered from asthma since being a kid but rarely experiences it now.

The above case brings up an important point; which is, whenever a meridian is added to complete a circuit, the patient should be questioned about any symptoms or history of conditions that pertain to that organ. Many times there will have been a history of imbalance in that system, and it is even common that the patient's fourth concern is directly related to that organ.

Case Study: Male, 63

Primary Complaint: Chronic left knee pain in the GB channel from GB 33 – GB 34

Secondary Complaint: Erectile Dysfunction – KI

Third Complaint: Congenital heart disease involving the mitral valve – HT

Tongue: Red and puffy with a thick yellow coat.

Pulse: Rapid and rolling.

This is a straight forward pattern in both circuit theory and zang-fu syndrome differentiation.

To construct the circuit we should recognize that the patient's primary concern involves the GB, which has a system two and four association with the heart.

GB - HT

We also know that his secondary and tertiary complaints involve the shao yin, and this allows us to add the KI to the developing circuit.

$$GB - HT$$
$$-$$
$$KI$$

To complete the circuit the SJ is added since it connects to both the GB and KI.

$$GB - HT$$
$$- \quad -$$
$$SJ - KI$$

Analyzing the case according to zang-fu methodologies the knee pain would be classified as Bi syndrome, or otherwise known as painful obstruction syndrome. In this disease the pathogenic factors are wind, cold, damp, heat, blood stasis, phlegm, liver and kidney deficiency. For his secondary concern of erectile dysfunction, the possible patterns are kidney deficiency and damp heat in the lower jiao. When all his signs and symptoms were taken into consideration the case was identified as a damp heat pattern.

Interesting enough his primary concern of knee pain was located from GB 33 – GB 34, and it is well known that GB 34 is commonly indicated for damp heat patterns. The points used on this case were right side: SJ 10, SJ 5, KI 3, KI 7, KI 9; and left side: HT 3, HT 7, and GB33.

Case Study: Female, 54

Primary Complaint: Right side wrist pain primarily on the PC and SJ meridians.

Secondary Concern: Headaches in the forehead and eyes that occur from eyestrain – LV and GB

Third Concern: Tight jaw with tension at GB 2 and GB 3.

The primary concern clearly involved the PC and SJ meridians. The pain was worse in the region of PC 6 - PC 7, and when severe she would feel the pain moving through the wrist to the SJ line. With this as the primary concern, it is appropriate to think of working with the PC - SJ meridian pair.

The secondary concern of headaches mostly occurred when she over used her eyes, and she would frequently feel the pain move from the eyes into the forehead. For headaches in the forehead it is common to think of the yang ming being involved, but it is always important to determine precisely where the pain is at. For this patient the pain would move from the eyes to the area near GB 14, and for this reason the secondary concern involved the LV - GB pair. The third concern of jaw tension was precisely located at GB 2 and GB 3, and both of these points were reactive to pressure.

Reviewing the patients top concerns we find the shao yang - jue yin circuit is able to account for all her symptoms.

The final point prescription included: right side SJ 3, SJ 5, LV 4, LV 3; Left side GB 40, 42, and PC 6.

Case Study: Male, 42

Primary Concern: Neck, back, and spinal pain along the UB and SI meridians. The pain was worse in the upper back and lumbar regions along both the inner and outer UB lines. At times there was pain in the SI meridian from the region of SI 10 – SI 15.

Secondary Concern: History of UB infections with clear and profuse urination.

Third Concern: Frequent loose stool that were worse with gluten, cheese, and dairy.

The patient also complained of low energy.

Tongue: Pale, slightly puffy, with small teeth marks.

From the primary and secondary concerns we can see an imbalance in the UB. The SI meridian is also involved in the primary concern, and for this reason the tai yang is the predominant pair to work with. From the third concern we see an obvious imbalance in the SP, and this was confirmed by the appearance of the tongue.

For this patient the tai yang - tai yin circuit was used with the addition of the KI meridian.

KI - UB - SI

\-   \-

LU - SP

The KI meridian was added because when the patient was asked about the history of the back and spinal pain, he indicated that there was a congenital condition that was contributing to it.   He had suffered from the pain since being a kid, and was told by numerous allopathic doctors that it was due to a birth defect. Since English was not his native language, it was impossible to get more information or a clear Western diagnosis about the nature of his spinal condition. Due to these reasons the KI meridian was added to the primary circuit. After eight treatments the patient frequently commented that his spine had never felt so good, and he became a source of many referrals.

Case Study: Female, 48

Main Concern: Chronic headaches in the GB meridian, fixed pain at GB 14 with pain and tenderness from GB20 - 21

Secondary Concern: Hot flashes from menopause – KI

Third Concern: Fatigue – KI, SP, HT, LU

Since the headaches were in the gallbladder meridian I first determined what meridians connect to the GB; these are the SJ, HT, and LV. The hot flashes were related to menopause and this pattern is associated with the kidney. From the client's main complaints I was anticipating a liver yang rising pattern with underlying kidney yin deficiency: I expected her tongue to be red and dry, but it was pale and puffy with teeth marks. The pulse was thin.

As I reviewed the patient's health history form there were numerous symptoms involving the spleen, and this also corresponded with her tongue presentations. A history of chronic anemia was confirmed, and I felt this was rooted in a spleen qi deficiency rather then some other etiological cause.

Based on the overall pattern, and the spleen's connection to the heart, the spleen was added to the circuit.

SJ - GB - LV
- -
SP/KI - HT

The presence of a liver yang rising pattern was apparent, but the tongue did not correspond with what was expected, especially with a secondary concern of menopausal hot flashes. As far as her third concern of fatigue, there were numerous possibilities that could be contributing to that. While it would have been possible to suppose that it was also resulting from the kidney deficiency, the numbers of spleen deficiency signs were in greater abundance than any other pattern. This led me to conclude that the liver yang rising, and temple headaches, were rooted in a kidney deficiency and heart-spleen blood deficiency. There was not enough yin and blood to keep the yang from rising to the head, nor was there enough blood in the vessels.

Case Study: Female, 30

Primary Complaint: Tightness in the chest with difficulty breathing. The symptoms were connected to her emotions and were worse with depression, sadness, and stress.

Secondary Concern: Depression and sadness connected to her family history.

With tightness in the chest there are several organs that could be responsible for the pattern. The lungs, heart, and liver could all be involved, and if it is a heart syndrome, the spleen and kidneys could also be contributing to the pattern. When the patient was asked about accompanying symptoms and the history of the condition, she expressed that it started during a particularly stressful time with her family. As a result of her family situation she frequently felt sadness, and she was well aware of a connection between her emotional state and the manifestation of her chest symptoms. When the tightness in the chest was present she had difficulty breathing, shortness of breath, and a suffocating sensation. Taking this into consideration the LU was taken to be a primary organ involved in the pattern.

For the purpose of doing a differential diagnosis the patient was asked about symptoms pertaining to a heart pattern. There were no heart signs such as palpitations, insomnia, stabbing pain, or radiating sensations in the shoulders or arm. The symptoms were not worse with exercise.

When asked about a third concern the patient stated she was very healthy and had no other symptoms to complain about. However, after inquiring with ten questions it was found that she occasionally suffered from headaches. They were located behind the eyes and were related to stress and overwork. Though the headaches were not a priority for her, she decided they were her third concern.

Since the primary concern was related to the lungs, and the third complaint was connected to the liver, the LU and LV were taken to be the primary meridian pair to work with. From a zang-fu perspective the pattern was identified as liver qi stagnation invading the lungs, and this allows us to begin to build a circuit using these two organs.

LU - LV

When reviewing the circuits that may be created with the LU - LV pair, we find that only the tai yang meridians of the UB and SI may be used to create a 4M circuit. However, these two meridians are not really pertinent to her pattern.

If we compare the five meridian systems of the LU and LV, we find that the LI connects to both of them. Since this is a liver qi stagnation pattern it is appropriate to use the LI meridian, and this allows us to form a circuit with these three channels.

LI
- -
LU - LV

As a final point prescription four gates was needled with thoracic four gates. That is LI 4, LV 3, LU 1, LV 14. The points were needled bilaterally, and after two treatments the symptoms resolved. A follow-up was done one year later, and the symptoms had not returned.

CHAPTER 11

COMPLETING THE CIRCLE

When doing syndrome differentiation according to circuit theory, there are two things that are essential for learning how to identify circuits of disharmony. The first is to know the five meridian systems for each of the 12 channels, and the second is to ask the patient about their top three health priorities. When these two techniques are used together it greatly assists the clinician in identifying zang-fu patterns and determining what circuits should be used. As a means to learn the systems and build circuits based on the patients needs, it is helpful to think of the meridians as pairs. This is common in conventional practices that often speak of the internal/external pairs and the six meridians.

The other pairings that are possible between the meridians are based on either the system two associations, or those generated from the horary cycle. This includes pairs such as the ST and PC, LU and UB, or the LI and KI.

By thinking in terms of meridians pairs we are able to have a much better understanding of disease etiology and pathogenesis. The various meridian pairs can also help us to understand branch and root patterns, and are beneficial for determining what meridians are most significant for treatment.

To aid us in clarifying our identification of zang-fu patterns and meridian circuits, the technique of asking the patient about their chief concerns is essential. Without doing this, the clinician may arrive at a diagnosis that inadequately accounts for the patient's most problematic symptoms. Though zang-fu patterns may be identified without asking the patient about their chief concerns, this method refines the diagnostic process and allows for more intelligent point combinations. When the clinician knows what symptoms are most significant to the patient, it simplifies working with complex patterns, and allows for greater precision in diagnosis and treatment.

At times it will be found that a patient may not have a tertiary, or even a secondary complaint, and in these cases there are several things that need to be considered. For some cases the primary concern will be so severe that secondary symptoms are seen as insignificant to the client. These people want relief from their primary concern, and any other symptoms they have may be of little consequence. For situations like this it is important to assure the client that their primary complaint will remain the focus of the treatment, but that it helps to know about any other symptoms that are present. Simply explain to them that knowing about these will give you a more holistic perspective, and allow you to do a better job. Clients are very responsive and appreciative to this type of explanation.

Another type of patient will be of such strong constitution that they are unable to come up with secondary complaints. Though many of these people do have other symptoms, they are so rarely felt, or of such minor degree, that the patient has a hard time commenting on them. For clients like this it is essential to do comprehensive intakes and ask about their health history. It is not uncommon when this is done that a client will reveal a symptom that they have infrequently, or at least recall something in their health history that is significant to their overall presentation.

Unilateral and Bilateral Needling

After the most relevant circuit has been identified in a patient's pattern, it is essential to determine how to apply the needles. For most cases I prefer unilateral needling, meaning that each point is only needled on one side of the body. This method is effective for all types of pain, and is especially important for acute conditions and traumatic injuries. This is because in acute conditions where there is tissue damage, needling into the traumatized area causes additional injury to the tissues and often makes the symptoms worse. If the affected meridian is treated, distal points from the pain should be chosen to avoid aggravating the injury any further.

Unilateral needling is also preferred when the patient has multiple patterns and a complex case. Whenever there is the presence of two or more zang-fu patterns, or if a 6M circuit is to be used, unilateral needling should be done so as to maximize the different points that can be used, while reducing the total number of points needled. For instance, suppose a patient has a primary complaint of headaches behind the eyes, a secondary concern of abdominal bloating, and a tertiary complaint of insomnia and dizziness. From a zang-fu perspective it is found that the patient has liver qi stagnation overacting on the spleen, with heart and spleen blood deficiency. The treatment strategy for this patient is to soothe the liver qi, strengthen the spleen, nourish the blood, and calm the shen. With such a complex pattern and extensive treatment strategy, it is possible to use too many needles when doing bilateral needling. If we were to needle LI 4, LV 3, PC 6, ST 36, SP 3, and SP 6 bilaterally, we would be using twelve needles.

Employing unilateral needling we could choose right side: LI 4, LI 10, LV 3, SP 3, SP 6 and left side: ST 36, PC 3, and PC 6. Doing this we have used only 8 needles, and are able to work with a greater variety of points. In summary, use unilateral needling when there are numerous symptoms with complex patterns, extensive pain, or in cases of acute and traumatic injuries.

For straightforward cases where there is only one zang-fu pattern present, or when a 4M circuit sufficiently addresses the patient's needs, bilateral needling may be preferred. When three or four meridians are all that needs to be treated, applying bilateral needling can effectively localize the therapy where it is most needed. For a case of spleen qi deficiency, where the chief concerns are all related to this pattern, bilateral needling is preferred because a limited number of meridians need to be needled. Bilateral needling is also indicated for many deficiency patterns, especially when there are only one or two organ systems involved.

The final decision to use unilateral or bilateral needling needs to be weighed using various factors. Generally speaking, complex patterns with diverse symptoms, excessive conditions, and pain are to be treated with unilateral needling; while bilateral needling is used for deficiencies, cases with one pattern, or when 2-4 meridians are sufficient to address the patient's condition. These are just general guidelines and each case needs to be accounted for individually.

A Final Note on Pattern Identification

In zang-fu pattern identification emphasis is placed on determining patterns of imbalance in the organ systems, and after this has been assessed, treatment strategies are determined and then meridians and points are selected.

In meridian circuit theory priority is placed on determining symptomatic meridians, assessing organ imbalances, and identifying 4M circuits. Once a 4M circuit has been identified, we may choose to add a meridian, or even a meridian pair, to the circuit to account for the patient's overall symptomatic expressions and root patterns. Thus, circuit theory bases syndrome differentiation on the 4M circuits, but it is also able to account for organ and 5-element imbalances. In this way, circuit theory includes the wisdom of 5-elements and zang-fu methods, but lends additional insight with its understanding of the connections that exist between the meridians. When circuit theory is part of the process of syndrome differentiation, it assists in refining both diagnosis and treatment, and this leads to greater clinical efficiency.

Dedicated to the Spirit Doctor
who is also known as the
Maroon Hummingbird.

Sources

1. Richard Tan, 2004, Lectures on the Balance Method and Master Tung's Points.

2. Wei-Chieh Young, 2008, Lectures on Tung's Acupuncture, American Chinese Medical Cultural Center.

3. Peter Deadman, Mazin Al-Khafaji, Kevin Baker, 2007, A Manual of Acupuncture, Journal of Chinese Medicine Publications.

4. Jeffrey Jacob, 1996, The Acupuncturist's Clinical Handbook, Aesclipius Press.

5. Maoshing Ni, 1995, The Yellow Emperor's Classic of Medicine, Shambhala.

6. Giovanni Maciocia, 1994, The Practice of Chinese Medicine, Churchill Livingstone.

For up to date information about publications, seminars, events, and international tours visit:

The Integrative Healing Society
www.ihsociety.com

Through his company, The Integrative Healing Society, James often leads tours to China, Thailand, Bali, Central America, and Peru. He also gives seminars throughout Europe and the United States, and he is widely recognized as a teacher of international standards.

Many of the tours and seminars he offers are accredited by the NCCAOM and NCBTMB for continuing education credits. For additional information about these tours and seminars you may write to him at:

james.spears@ihsociety.com

CPSIA information can be obtained at www.ICGtesting.com
Printed in the USA
LVOW011342140911

246268LV00005B/14/P

9 781453 784204